A clinical guide to orthodontics

A clinical guide to orthodontics

Dai Roberts-Harry MSc, FDS, MOrth
Orthodontic Department, Leeds Dental Institute, Clarendon Way, Leeds, LS2 9LU

Jonathan R Sandy PhD, FDS, MOrth
Division of Child Dental Health, University of Bristol Dental School,
Lower Maudlin Street, Bristol, BS1 2LY

2003
Published by the British Dental Association
64 Wimpole Street, London, W1G 8YS

Preface

This book intends to draw together some of the main issues in orthodontics which are of relevance to students, general dental practitioners and orthodontists. As the number of orthodontic trainees increases, there may be enough specialist practitioners to cater for most of the UK's orthodontic care, provided there is appropriate referral.

Where then does the general dental practitioner fit into this scenario? There will always be a number of general dental practitioners who have a specific interest in orthodontics and who, through enthusiasm and commitment, will acquire orthodontic treatment skills. With increasing specialisation in many areas, one of the biggest burdens on general dental practitioners will be appropriate diagnosis and subsequent referral.

This book tries to tease out the key issues in orthodontics and the specific areas that do need action during the development of the occlusion. It also attempts to show a broad range of current orthodontic options and highlights some of the pitfalls associated with treatment.

The authors were both undergraduates at a dental school, which at the time was famous for not inspiring orthodontic students! Both have different clinical and academic skills but found orthodontics a difficult concept as undergraduates, so much so that postgraduate education was the only way that either could grasp this complex subject. Therefore, we hope that this book will have some value for the students who also find this a tricky area.

Acknowledgements

The authors are grateful to their colleagues who provided encouragement and guidance in the preparation of this book. Many of the ideas and concepts in the text are not our own but have been assimilated from a multitude of clinicians and academic staff too numerous to specifically mention. We are also grateful to a number of secretarial staff who have helped us.

D Roberts-Harry
J R Sandy
November 2003

ISBN 0 904588 78 5 softback
ISBN 0 904588 81 5 hardback

Printed and bound by
Dennis Barber Limited, Lowestoft, Suffolk

Contents

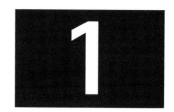

IN BRIEF

- This series of articles is designed to aid in the orthodontic evaluation of patients
- Not every malocclusion needs orthodontic treatment
- Not every patient is suitable for treatment
- Understanding the treatment benefit for the patient is important
- GDPs have an important role to play in assessing the need for orthodontic treatment

Who needs orthodontics?

D. Roberts-Harry and J. Sandy

There are various reasons for offering patients orthodontic treatment. Some of these include improved aesthetics, occlusal function and long-term dental health.

Orthodontics comes from the Greek words 'orthos' meaning normal, correct, or straight and 'dontos' meaning teeth. Orthodontics is concerned with correcting or improving the position of teeth and correcting any malocclusion. What then do we mean by occlusion and malocclusion? Surprisingly the answer is not straightforward. There have been various attempts to describe occlusion using terms such as ideal, anatomic (based on tooth morphology), average, aesthetic, adequate, normally functioning and occlusion unlikely to impair dental health.

With these different definitions of what constitutes malocclusion, there is, not surprisingly a degree of confusion as to what should be treated and what should not. Although some tooth positions can produce tooth and soft tissue trauma, it is important to remember that malocclusion is not a disease but simply a variation in the normal position of teeth. Essentially, there are three principal reasons for carrying out orthodontic treatment:

1. To improve dento facial appearance
2. To correct the occlusal function of the teeth

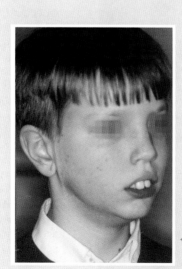

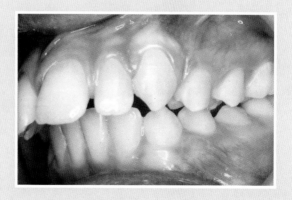

Fig. 1a A child with a Class II division 1 malocclusion and very poor aesthetic appearance

Fig. 1b The same child as in Fig. 1a

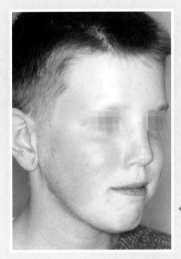

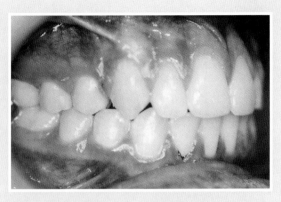

◀ Fig. 2a Same child as in Fig. 1 after orthodontic treatment

▲ Fig. 2b Occlusion of the same patient as in Fig. 2a, there has been a significant improvement in the buccal segment relation and overjet compared with the initial presentation in Fig. 1b

Table 1 Features children most dislike or are teased about (Shaw et al.[1])

Feature	Disliked appearance or teased (%)
Teeth	60.7
Clothes	53.8
Ears	51.7
Weight	41.5
Brace	33.3
Nose	29.3
Height	25.3

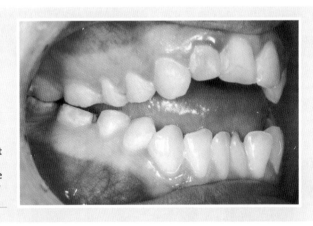

Fig. 3 This patient has a severe anterior open bite with contact only on the molars

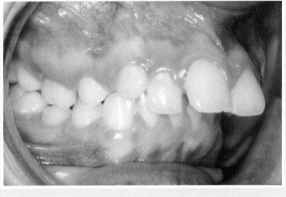

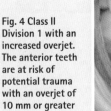

Fig. 4 Class II Division 1 with an increased overjet. The anterior teeth are at risk of potential trauma with an overjet of 10 mm or greater

3. To eliminate occlusion that could damage the long-term health of the teeth and periodontium

DENTO FACIAL APPEARANCE

Improving the appearance of the teeth is without question the main reason why most orthodontic treatment is undertaken. Although it might be tempting to dismiss this as a trivial need, there is little doubt that a poor dental appearance can have a profound psychosocial effect on children. Figure 1 illustrates such a case with a child who has a substantial aesthetic need for treatment. The case is shown before (Fig. 1a, b) and after (Fig 2a, b) orthodontic treatment. Few would question that there has been an improvement in both the dental and facial appearance of this child. Indeed, orthodontic treatment can have a beneficial psychosocial effect. For example Shaw et al.[1] found that children were teased more about their teeth than anything else, such as the clothes they wear or their weight and height (Table 1).

OCCLUSAL FUNCTION

Teeth, which do not occlude properly, can make eating difficult and may predispose to temporomandibular joint (TMJ) dysfunction. However, the association with TMJ dysfunction and malocclusion is a controversial subject and will be discussed in more detail in a later section. Individuals who have poor occlusion, such as shown in Figure 3, may find it difficult and embarrassing to eat because they cannot bite through food using their incisors. They can only chew food using their posterior teeth.

DENTAL HEALTH

Surprisingly there is no strong association between dental irregularity and dental caries or periodontal disease. It seems that dietary factors are much more important than the alignment of the teeth in the aetiology of caries. Although straight teeth may be easier to clean than crooked ones, patient motivation and dental hygiene seems to be the overriding factor in preventing gingivitis and periodontitis. That said, few of the studies that have investigated the link between crowding and periodontal disease have been longitudinal, over a long term and included older adults. It would appear that aligned teeth confer no benefit to those who clean their teeth well because they can keep their teeth clean regardless of any irregularity. Similarly, alignment will not help bad brushers. If there is poor tooth brushing, periodontal diseases will develop no matter how straight the teeth are. However, having straight teeth may help moderate brushers, although there is no firm evidence to support or refute this statement. This is an area that requires further study.

Some malocclusions may damage both the teeth and soft tissues if they are left untreated. It is well known that the more prominent the upper incisors are the more prone they are to trauma[2,3] (Table 2).

When the overjet is 9 mm or more the risk of damaging the upper incisors increases to over 40%. Reducing a large overjet is not only beneficial from an aesthetic point of view but minimises the risk of trauma and long-term complications to the dentition. Fig. 4 shows a child with a large overjet and it is not difficult to imagine the likely dental trauma that would result if he or she fell over.

Table 2 Relation between size of overjet and prevalence of traumatised anterior teeth

Overjet (mm)	Incidence %
5	22
9	24
>9	44

Certain other occlusal relationships are also liable to cause long-term problems. Figure 5a and b show a case where there is an anterior cross-bite with an associated mandibular displacement in a 60-year-old man. The constant attrition of the lower incisors against the upper when the patient bites together, have produced some substantial wear. If allowed to continue then the long-term prognosis for these teeth is extremely poor. In order to preserve the teeth, the patient accepted fixed appliance treatment that eliminated the cross bite and helped prevent further wear Figure 5c and d.

Another example of problems caused by an anterior cross bite is shown in Figure 6. A traumatic anterior occlusion produced a displacing force on the lower incisors with apical migration of the gingival attachment as a consequence. Provided this situation is remedied early (Fig. 7) the soft tissue damage stops and as the rest of the gingivae matures the situation often resolves

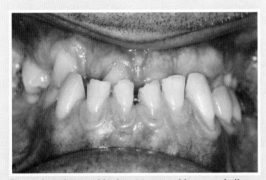

Fig. 5a Anterior crossbite in a 60-year-old man occluding in the intercuspal position

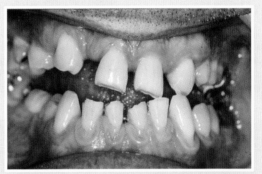

Fig. 5b Shows the retruded contact position of the patient. To reach full intercuspation the mandible displaces forward and this movement is probably associated with the wear on the incisors

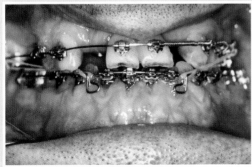

Fig. 5c The patient in fixed appliances in order to correct the displacement and the position of his upper anterior teeth

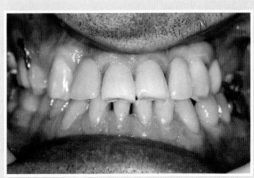

Fig. 5d After correction and space reorganisation the patient is wearing a prosthesis to replace the missing lateral incisors

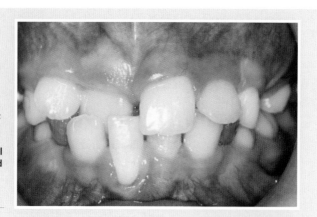

Fig. 6 A traumatic anterior occlusion is displacing the lower right central incisor labially and there is an associated dehiscence

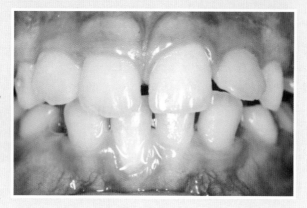

Fig. 7 The same patient as in Fig. 6, but the cross bite has been corrected with a removable appliance and there has been an improvement in the gingival condition

vidual will receive from this will depend on the severity of the presenting malocclusion as well as the patient's own perception of the problem. Some individuals can have a marked degree of dento-facial deformity and be unconcerned with their appearance. Although a practitioner may suggest treatment for such an individual, patients should not be talked into treatment and must be left to make the final decision themselves. Mild malocclusions should be treated with caution. Not only will the net improvement in the appearance of the teeth be small, but also as nearly all teeth move to some degree after orthodontic treatment the risk of relapse in these cases is high. Whilst minor movements after the correction of severe malocclusions will still produce a substantial net overall improvement for the patients, the same is not true of minor problems. Many practitioners will have encountered the parent who can spot a 5-degree rotation of an upper lateral incisor from fifty metres and is convinced this will be the social death of their child. Regardless of how insistent the parent or child is, the practitioner should approach such problems

spontaneously and no long-term problems usually develop.

Deep overbites can occasionally cause stripping of the soft tissues as shown in Figure 8a and b. This is a case where there is little aesthetic need for treatment but because of the deep overbite there is substantial damage to the soft tissues. Clearly if this is allowed to continue there is a risk of early loss of the lower incisors that would produce a difficult restorative problem.

WHO SHOULD BE TREATED?

Dental irregularity alone is not an indication for treatment. Most orthodontic treatment is carried out for aesthetic reasons and the benefit an indi-

Table 3 Index of Treatment Need

Dental health component	Treatment need
1	No need
2	Little need
3	Moderate need
4	Great need
5	Very great need

Aesthetic component	Treatment need
1	
2	Little need
3	
4	
5	
6	Moderate need
7	
8	
9	Great need
10	

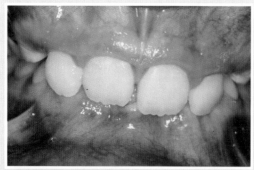

Fig. 8a This malocclusion has an extremely deep bite which can be associated with potential periodontal problems

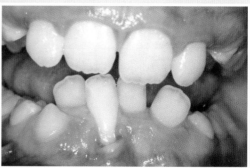

Fig. 8b The same patient as in Fig. 8a, but not in occlusion. The deep bite has resulted in labial stripping of the periodontium on the lower right central incisor

with care and only carry out the treatment if it is in the best interests of the patient. It is essential that the patient and parent are fully aware of the limitations of treatment and that long term, ie permanent retention is currently the only way to ensure long-term alignment of the teeth.

In order to assess the need for orthodontic treatment, various indices have been developed. The one used most commonly in the United Kingdom is the Index of Orthodontic Treatment Need (IOTN).[4] This index attempts to rank malocclusion, in order, from worst to best. It comprises two parts, an aesthetic component and a dental health component (Table 3). The aesthetic component consists of a series of ten photographs ranging from most to least attractive. The idea is to match the patient's malocclusion as closely as possible with one of the photographs. It is unlikely that a perfect match will be found but the practitioner should use his or her best guess to match to the nearest equivalent photograph. The dental health component consists of a series of occlusal traits that could affect the long-term dental health of the teeth. Various features are graded from 1–5 (least severe – worst). The worst feature of the presenting malocclusion is matched to the list and given the appropriate score.

Many hospital orthodontic services will not accept patients in categories 1–3 of the dental health component or grade 6 or less of the aesthetic component of the IOTN unless they are suitable for undergraduate teaching purposes.

Whilst the IOTN is a useful guide in prioritising treatment and determining treatment need it

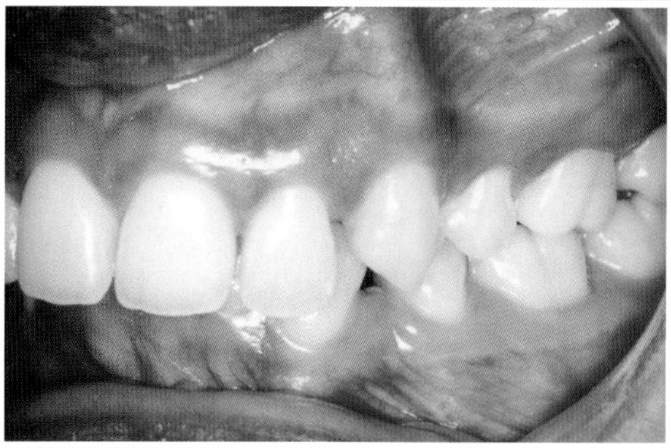

Fig. 9 The Index of Treatment Need for this patient is 2. Although this is low, the level of expertise required to treat it is high

takes no account of the degree of treatment difficulty. For example, class II division 2 malocclusions are notoriously difficult to treat yet they might have a low IOTN. Figure 9 illustrates such a case. The IOTN of this patient is only 2 but it is a difficult case to manage and treatment requires a high level of expertise.

1. Shaw W C, Meek S C, Jones D S. Nicknames, teasing, harassment and the salience of dental features among school children. *Br J Orthod* 1980; **7:** 75-80.
2. Office of Population Censuses and Surveys (1994). *Children's dental health in the United Kingdom 1993.* London: HMSO 0116916079.
3. Office of Population Censuses and Surveys (1985). *Children's dental health in the United Kingdom 1983.* London: HMSO 0116911360.
4. Brook P, Shaw W C. The development of an index of orthodontic treatment priority. *Eur J Orthod* 1989; **11:** 309-320.

IN BRIEF

- Careful patient assessment is the most important part of treatment
- The extra-oral examination is conducted first
- The skeletal relationship must be assessed three-dimensionally
- The teeth lie in a position of soft tissue balance
- Habits such as thumb sucking can induce a malocclusion
- There is no proven association between TMJ dysfunction and orthodontics

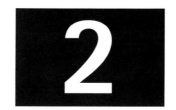

Patient assessment and examination I

D. Roberts-Harry and J. Sandy

The patient assessment forms the essential basis of orthodontic treatment. This is divided into an extra-oral and intra-oral examination. The extra-oral examination is carried out first as this can fundamentally influence the treatment options. The skeletal pattern, soft tissue form and the presence or absence of habits must all be taken into account.

The most important part of orthodontic treatment is the patient assessment. Once a particular treatment strategy is started subsequent changes are often difficult. If it is decided that extractions are needed and since the process is irreversible, they must be carefully considered in the treatment planning process. Inappropriate orthodontic treatment can produce adverse results and it is essential that full examination of skeletal form, soft tissue relationships and occlusal features are performed prior to undertaking treatment. It is sensible to carry out the assessment in a logical order so that none of the steps are missed. A simple assessment should include the following:

- Medical history
- Patient's complaint
- Extra-oral examination
- Intra-oral examination
- Radiographs
- Orthodontic indices
- Justification for treatment
- Treatment aims
- Treatment plan

This section concentrates on the extra- and intra-oral examination of the patient.

EXTRA–ORAL EXAMINATION

It is helpful to follow the examination sequence outlined:

- Skeletal pattern
- Soft tissues
- Temporomandibular joint examination

Skeletal pattern

Patients are three-dimensional and therefore the skeletal pattern must be assessed in anterior-posterior (A-P), vertical and transverse relationships. Although the soft tissues can tip the crowns of the teeth the skeletal pattern fundamentally determines their apical root position. The relative size of the mandible and maxilla to each other will determine the skeletal pattern. The smaller the mandible or the larger the maxilla the more the patient will be Class II. Conversely with a bigger mandible or smaller maxilla the patient will be more Class III. The bigger the size discrepancy between the maxilla and mandible, the more difficult treatment becomes and the less likely it is that orthodontics alone will be able to correct the malocclusion. Although some orthodontic appliances have a small orthopaedic effect, treatment is generally most easily accomplished on patients with a normal skeletal pattern and a normal relationship of the maxilla to the mandible.

Anterior–posterior (AP)

Although precise skeletal relationships can be determined using a lateral cephalostat radiograph, many practices do not have this facility and it is important to be able to assess the skeletal relationships clinically.

To assess the AP skeletal pattern the patient has to be postured carefully with the head in a neutral horizontal position (Frankfort Plane horizontal to the floor). Different head postures can mask the true relationship. If the head is tipped back the chin tends to come further forward and makes the patient appear to be more Class III.

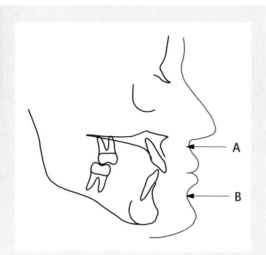

Fig. 1
A tracing of
a lateral cephalostat
radiograph identifying soft
tissue points A and B

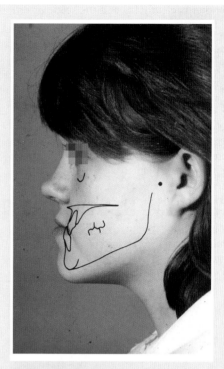

Fig. 2 Shows a patient with a skeletal III pattern where a tracing of the lateral cephalostat radiograph has been superimposed on the photograph. The soft tissue masks to some extent a significant skeletal III pattern

Conversely, if the head is tipped down the chin moves back and the patient appears to be more Class II. Sit the patient upright in the dental chair and ask them to occlude gently on their posterior teeth. Ask them to gaze at a distant point; this will usually bring them into a fairly neutral horizontal head position. Look at the patient in profile and identify the most concave points on the soft tissue profile of the upper and lower lips (Fig. 1).

The point on the upper lip is called soft tissue A point and on the lower lip soft tissue B point. In a patient with a class I skeletal pattern B point is situated approximately 1 mm behind A point. The further back B point is, the more the pattern is skeletal II and the more anterior, the more skeletal III it becomes. Figure 2 shows a patient with a skeletal III pattern where the outline of the hard tissues has been superimposed on the photograph. This demonstrates that although we are examining the soft tissue outline this also gives an indication of the

underlying skeletal pattern. Obviously the soft tissue thickness may vary and mask the A–P skeletal pattern to some degree but generally the thickness of the upper and lower lips is similar. The underlying skeletal pattern is therefore often reflected in the soft tissue pattern. The more severe the skeletal pattern is the more difficult treatment of the resulting malocclusion becomes. Figure 3a and b, shows an adult with an obvious skeletal III pattern and a malocclu-

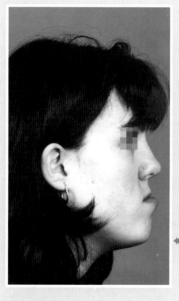

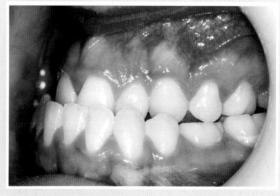

◀ Fig. 3a Profile of an adult who has an obvious skeletal III pattern

⬆ Fig. 3b Malocclusions of the same patient in Figure 3a. The patient has a Class III malocclusion which is beyond the scope of orthodontics alone

sion that is clearly beyond the scope of orthodontic treatment alone.

Vertical dimension

This dimension gives some indication of the degree of overbite. The vertical dimension is usually measured in terms of facial height and the shorter the anterior facial height the more likely it is that the patient will have a deep overbite. Conversely the longer the facial height the more the patient is likely to have an anterior open bite. Deep overbites associated with a short anterior facial height and open bites with long face heights are difficult to correct with orthodontics alone. The greater the skeletal difference the more likely it is that the patient will need a combination of orthodontics and orthognathic surgery to correct the occlusion and the underlying skeletal discrepancy.

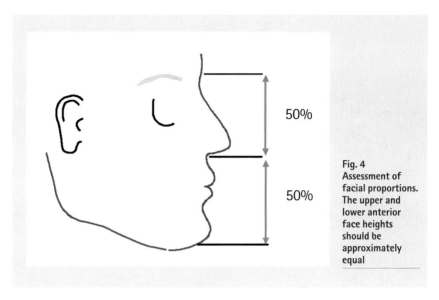

Fig. 4
Assessment of facial proportions. The upper and lower anterior face heights should be approximately equal

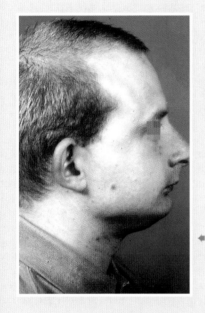

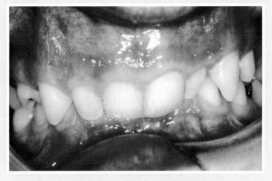

◄▥ Fig. 5 Profile of a patient with a much reduced lower anterior facial height

⬆ Fig. 6 Occlusion of the patient shown in Figure 5. The reduced lower anterior face height is often associated with a deep bite as shown

There are various ways of measuring the vertical dimension, one of the most common is to measure the Frankfort Mandibular Planes Angle. This is not a very easy clinical angle to measure and the problem is compounded by the fact that not many clinicians can identify the Frankfort Plane correctly. A more practical way of assessing this is simply to measure the vertical dimension as indicated in Figure 4.

The lower anterior facial height is the distance from the base of the chin to the base of the nose. The upper anterior facial height is the distance from the base of the nose to a point roughly between the eyebrows. These dimensions can be measured with a ruler although the index finger and thumb will do almost as well. The lower and upper facial heights are usually equal. If the lower anterior facial height is reduced, as illustrated in Figure 5, this can result in a deep overbite that can be difficult to correct (Fig. 6). Conversely, if the lower anterior facial height is greater

than 50% this can produce an anterior openbite (Fig. 7).

Transverse dimension

To assess this dimension, look at the patient head-on and assess whether there is any asym-

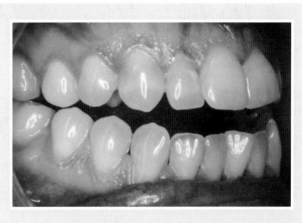

Fig. 7 Anterior open bites are often associated with an increase in lower anterior face height

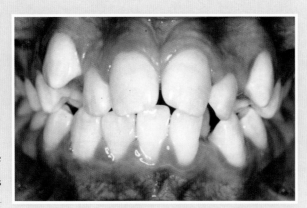

Fig. 8 A centre line shift where the lower centre line is to the left

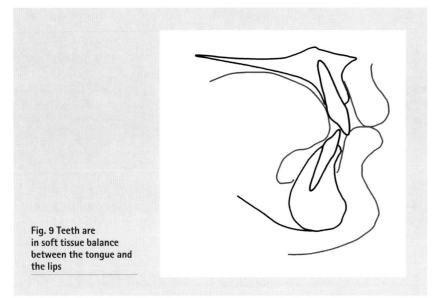

Fig. 9 Teeth are in soft tissue balance between the tongue and the lips

Fig. 10 These diagrams show how partial reduction of the overjet does not allow the lip to cover the upper incisors. The upper incisors are then quite likely to return to their pre-treatment position

metry in the facial mid-line. If there appears to be any mandibular asymmetry this may be reflected in the position of the teeth as shown in Fig. 8. If there is asymmetry it is important to distinguish between false and true asymmetry. A false asymmetry arises when occlusal interferences force the patient to displace the mandible laterally producing a cross-bite in the anterior or buccal region. If the displacement is eliminated then the mandible will return to a centric position. A true asymmetry arises as a consequence of unequal facial growth on the left or right side of the jaws. In these cases elimination of any occlusal cross-bites (which can be very difficult) is unlikely to improve the facial asymmetry.

SOFT TISSUE EXAMINATION

The soft tissues comprise the lips, cheeks and tongue and these guide the crowns of the teeth into position as they erupt. Ultimately, the teeth will lie in a position of soft tissue balance between the tongue on one side and the lips and cheeks on the other (Fig. 9).

In patients with a Class I incisor relationship the soft tissues rarely play an important part unless there is an anterior open-bite. The anterior open-bite may be caused by a digit sucking habit, a large lower anterior facial height, localised failure of eruption of the teeth, proclination of the incisors or to an endogenous tongue thrust. The latter cause is very rare and is usually identified by a large thrusting tongue that seems to permanently sit between the upper and lower incisors. This type of anterior open-bite is extremely difficult to correct. It is usually possible to reduce it, but on completion of treatment the tongue invariably pushes between the teeth and they move apart once again.

An important aspect of lip position is seen in patients with an increased overjet. If the upper incisor prominence is reduced, stability usually depends on the lower lip covering the upper incisors in order to prevent the overjet increasing post-treatment. Therefore, careful examination of the position of the lower lip in relation to the upper incisors is important. If the lower lip does not cover the upper incisors sufficiently after treatment, relapse of the overjet may occur. Similarly, if the overjet is to be reduced, full reduction is very important in order to give the lip the best possible chance of stabilising the incisors. Figure 10 illustrates the point; partial reduction of the overjet does not allow the lip to cover the upper incisors and they are likely to return to their pre-treatment position.

Whilst many young children have incompetent lips, this is often just a normal stage of development. As they pass through puberty, the lip length increases relative to the size of the face and the degree of lip competence gradually improves (Fig. 11).[1]

Lip incompetence can be caused by either a lack of lip tissue or an adverse skeletal pattern. If

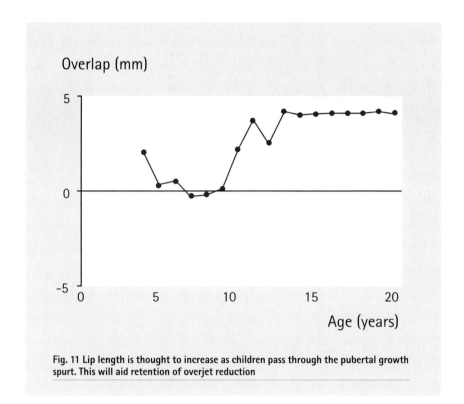

Fig. 11 Lip length is thought to increase as children pass through the pubertal growth spurt. This will aid retention of overjet reduction

the skeletal pattern is unfavourable in either the vertical or anterior-posterior position then even with normal lip length the soft tissues are still widely separated.

HABITS

Digit sucking is a well-known factor in producing anterior open-bite, proclined upper incisors and buccal cross-bites. If the habit ceases while the child is still growing then the incisors are very likely to return to their normal position. However, once the teenage years are passed and facial growth slows down, spontaneous resolution becomes increasingly unlikely. If the habit persists into adult life it may be necessary to use appliance treatment to correct the habit induced anterior open-bite. Buccal cross-bite possibly produced by digit sucking habits, rarely resolve spontaneously on cessation of the habit because of occlusal interferences. These buccal cross-bites often

need to be corrected with active appliance treatment.

TEMPORO-MANDIBULAR JOINT PROBLEMS

A comprehensive review of the literature by Luther[2,3] failed to demonstrate any conclusive association between TMJ dysfunction, malocclusion and orthodontic treatment. However, it is important that the joints are palpated and assessed for signs and symptoms of TMJ dysfunction. Patients who present with TMJ pain seeking an orthodontic solution to correct the problems should be treated with caution.

1. Vig P S, Cohen A M. Vertical growth of the lips: a serial cephalometric study. *Am J Orthod* 1979; **75:** 405-415.
2. Luther F. Orthodontics and the tempromandibular joint: where are we now? Part 1. Orthodontic treatment and temporomandibular disorders. *Angle Orthod* 1998; **68:** 305-318.
3. Luther F. Orthodontics and the temporomandibular joint: where are we now? Part 2. Functional occlusion, malocclusion, and TMD. *Angle Orthod* 1998; **68:** 305-318.

IN BRIEF
- Careful patient assessment is the most important part of treatment
- The intra-oral examination is conducted after the extra-oral assessment
- The degree of occlusal discrepancy influences the treatment options
- The dental health and patient motivation determine if appliance therapy can be used

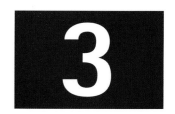

Patient assessment and examination II

D. Roberts-Harry and J. Sandy

The intra-oral assessment examines the oral health, individual tooth positions and inter-occlusal relationships. When this has been completed in conjunction with the extra-oral examination, a treatment plan can then be formulated.

INTRA–ORAL EXAMINATION

There are various systems available to assess this aspect but the following sequence is both practical and thorough:

- Dental health
- Lower arch
- Upper arch
- Teeth in occlusion
- Radiographs

Dental health

Even individuals with severe malocclusions should not have active orthodontic treatment in the presence of dental disease. Orthodontic appliances accumulate plaque and if the patient has a poor diet and tooth brushing then irreversible damage can result as demonstrated in Figure 1. Although the patient has straight teeth there is considerable decalcification and it could be argued is worse off as a consequence of treatment. Clearly this could have serious medicolegal complications, particularly if the clinician fails to write in the notes that appropriate dental health advice has been given

Decalcification around orthodontic appliances is a recognised hazard and will occur in the presence of poor oral hygiene and a cariogenic diet. Not only will decalcification occur around the brackets but tooth movement in the presence of active gingivitis or periodontal disease will accelerate any bone loss. Attempting to move teeth in the presence of active dental disease can have disastrous consequences and must be avoided.

Therefore, treatment for patients with ques-tionable dental health should be confined to extractions and spontaneous alignment of the teeth only. Figure 2 illustrates a case where there is an obvious need for orthodontic treatment but this was precluded by the patient's extremely poor oral hygiene.

Minor apical root resorption is a common consequence of orthodontic tooth movement. However, this resorption can occasionally be severe. Tooth movement in the presence of apical pathology is known to accelerate resorption and should be dealt with prior to commencing treatment.

Lower arch

The lower arch should be examined and planned in the first instance. Whatever treatment is carried out in the lower arch often determines the treatment to be carried out in the upper. Examine the teeth for any tipping, rotations and crowding. Teeth which are tipped mesially are much more amenable to treatment, both with removable and fixed appliances than teeth which are distally tipped. They also respond much better to extractions and spontaneous alignment than other teeth. The presence or absence of rotations is important because rotated teeth are most easily treated with fixed appliances. The more crowded the teeth are the more likely it is that extractions will be needed in order to correct the malocclusion. A method of assessing crowding is given in Figure 3. Firstly, measure the size of the teeth and add these together (length A). Then measure from the mid-line to the distal of the canine with a pair of dividers. Measure from the distal of the canine to the mesial of the first permanent

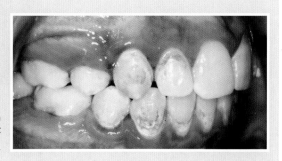

Fig. 1 Decalcification attributable to fixed appliances and a patient with poor oral hygiene throughout treatment

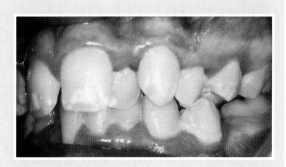

Fig. 2 This patient has a reasonable need for orthodontic treatment, but the poor oral hygiene and gingival condition precludes this

Upper arch

This is examined in a similar way to the lower arch. Additional points to note in the mixed dentition are the presence of a mid-line diastema and the position of the upper canines.

A mid-line diastema is commonly seen in the mixed dentition. The aetiological factors to be considered are:

- Normal (physiological) development
- Fraenum
- Small teeth
- Missing teeth
- Midline supernumerary

Physiologic spacing usually disappears as the occlusion matures, especially when the upper permanent canines erupt and no treatment apart from observation is needed. Fraenectomies are rarely indicated and generally do not need to be removed unless the fraenum is particularly large and fleshy.

The upper permanent canine should be palpable in the buccal sulcus by 10 years of age. If not, and the deciduous canine is firm, parallax radiography should be undertaken to determine where the permanent tooth is. If the tooth is palatally positioned then the deciduous canines on both sides should be removed. This will help guide the permanent tooth into a more favourable path of eruption and prevent any centre line shift caused by a unilateral deciduous extraction. It is essential that this palpation be carried out on all patients in this age group. Very often impacting canines are missed and the patient not referred for treatment until 15 or 16 years of age. Not only is this negligent, but the patient may then need to undergo a lengthy course of treatment at a socially difficult time.

Teeth in occlusion

The overjet and overbite should be measured and the incisor classification assessed. The British Standards Institute (BS EN21942 Part 1 (1992) Glossary of Dental terms) defines the incisor classification as follows:

molar. Add these together to give you the approximate arch length (length B). Subtract B from A to give you the degree of crowding. This must be repeated for both sides of the arch.

The degree of crowing influences the need for extractions. Although one should not be dogmatic and several other factors influence the planning of extractions, as a general rule the greater the crowding the more likely extractions are necessary. Table 1 gives an outline of the relation between degree of crowding and need for extractions.

Table 1 Relationship between crowding and extractions

Degree of crowding	Need for extractions
< 5 mm	No
5–10 mm	Possibly
> 10 mm	Yes

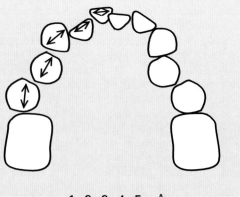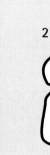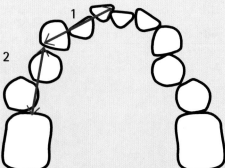

Fig. 3 Assessment of crowding. The widths of all the teeth anterior to the molars are measured and subtracted from the sum of two measurements (mesial of the lower incisor to the distal of the lower canine, plus distal of lower canine to the mesial of the first molar) to give the degree of crowding

1+2+3+4+5 = A

1+2 = B

B – A = Degree of crowding

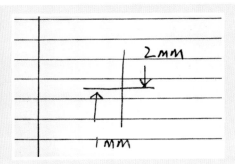

Fig. 5 Method for recording deviations in the centre line where the lower is to the right by 1mm and the upper to the left by 2 mm

- *Class I*. The lower incisor edges occlude with or lie immediately below the cingulum plateau (middle part of) the upper central incisors.
- *Class II*. The lower incisor edges lie posterior to the cingulum plateau of the upper central incisors. There are two divisions:
  Division 1 – there is an increase in the overjet and the upper central incisors are usually proclined.
  Division 2 – the upper central incisors are retroclined. The overjet is usually minimal but may be increased.
- *Class III*. The lower incisor edges lie anterior to the cingulum plateau of the upper central incisors. The overjet is reduced or reversed.

The centre line should be measured by placing a ruler down the patient's facial mid-line and measuring how far away from this the centre lines deviate (Fig. 4). This can then be marked in the notes as shown in Figure 5.

The buccal occlusion is assessed next, particularly the molar relationship. This is important because when assessing the treatment, it has to be decided whether the buccal occlusion is to be accepted or whether it should be corrected as part of the treatment plan. The canine and molar relationships should be recorded as class I, II or III

Finally, the presence of any anterior or posterior cross-bites should be assessed and if there is a cross-bite, the clinician should check to see whether there is any mandibular displacement associated with it. This is important because any displacement will mask the position of the teeth and give a misleading indication of the inter-occlusal relationships. Figure 6 shows a child who has an apparently severe class III incisor relationship. However, he can get his teeth into an edge-to-edge relationship and in this position the occlusion does not appear to be so severe. The amount of proclination of the upper incisors needed to correct the incisor relationship was quite mild and easily accomplished using a removable appliance (Fig. 7 and 8).

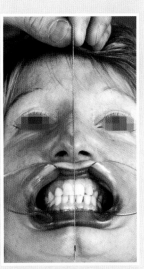

Fig. 4 Measurement of centre line deviation using a ruler placed in the patient's mid line

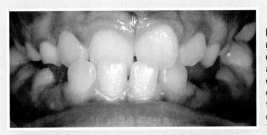

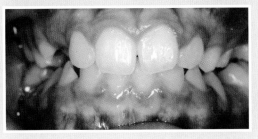

Fig. 6 Class III malocclusion with a displacement anteriorly. The patient can achieve an edge to edge incisor relation in the retruded position of the mandible

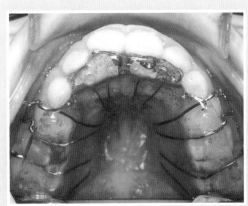

Fig. 7 Upper removable appliance used to correct the anterior cross bite

Fig. 8 The corrected incisor position for the patient

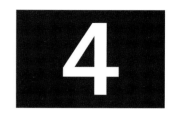
IN BRIEF

- Treatment planning is an essential part of orthodontic management
- Consider the Treatment Aims first, then the Treatment Plan
- The teeth and periodontium must be healthy before starting orthodontic treatment
- To help ensure a successful treatment outcome the oral hygiene and diet must be good
- Choosing the correct appliance is important

Treatment planning

D. Roberts-Harry and J. Sandy

The treatment plan is an integral part of orthodontic management. It should be divided into both treatment aims (what do you want to do?) and plan (how are you going to do it?). The treatment aims will include, for example overjet reduction. The plan will consider how to create space in order to accomplish this as well as the appliance system that will be used.

Treatment planning is the second most important part of orthodontic management following the patient examination. It is helpful to divide treatment planning into two sections, Treatment Aims and Treatment Plan. Although it is possible that orthodontic treatment can influence the skeletal form when growth-modifying (functional) appliances are used, it has little effect on soft tissues, tooth size and arch length. Remember that it is not necessary to treat every malocclusion and the benefits to the patient should be carefully assessed prior to undertaking any orthodontic treatment.

TREATMENT AIMS
The following list is not comprehensive and has to be tailored to the individual case. Some of the problems that may need to be addressed during treatment are:

- Improve dental health
- Relieve crowding
- Correct the buccal occlusion
- Reduce the overbite
- Reduce the overjet
- Align the teeth

As emphasised previously, it is essential that the oral health is of a high standard before treatment starts. Carious teeth should be restored and the periodontal condition and oral hygiene should be excellent before treatment starts.

Relieve crowding
The decision to extract teeth needs to be carefully considered and depends on the degree of crowding, the difficulty of the case and the degree of overbite correction.

Correct the buccal occlusion
The key to upper arch alignment is to get the canines into a Class I relationship (Fig. 1).

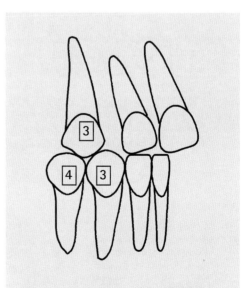

Fig. 1 It is important to achieve a Class I canine position in order to fully correct the overjet and the buccal segment relations

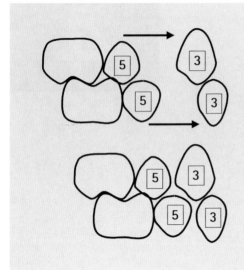

Fig. 2 The importance of keeping extraction patterns symmetrical is demonstrated. The lower arch crowding has been dealt with by removal of two lower premolars. The loss of the corresponding upper premolars means the molar relationship at the end of treatment should be Class I

Providing the lower incisors are well aligned, achieving this will generally produce sufficient space to align the upper incisors.

In order to get the canines Class I there are, in general two choices for the molar relationship at the end of treatment; either Class I or a full unit Class II. This will be covered in more detail later in the section on treatment plan.

Overbite and overjet reduction
The overbite should always be reduced before overjet reduction is attempted. A deep overbite will physically prevent the overjet from being reduced because of contact between the upper and lower incisors.

Retention
Once the overjet has been reduced and or upper incisors have been aligned a retainer should be fitted. These are designed to reduce the risk of relapse post treatment by allowing remodelling and consolidation of the alveolar bone around the teeth and reorganisation and maturation of the periodontal fibres. There are many different types of retainers but they are generally removable or fixed. There are no hard and fast rules regarding the length of time retention should continue. The authors recommend for removable appliance treatment that retention should continue for 3 months full time and 3 months at night-time only. For fixed appliance cases this should be 3 months full time and a minimum of 9 months at night-time only. At the end of this minimum year's worth of retention, discretionary wear should be advised. This means that the patient is given the option of discarding the retainer if they are fed up with wearing it, or continuing on a part-time regime to give the teeth the best possible chance of staying straight. If they decide to stop wearing the retainer they should be warned there is no guarantee that the teeth will remain straight throughout life and the only way to improve this prospect is by indefinite (ie life-long) wearing of the retainer.

Some cases especially those that were spaced or where rotations were present prior to treatment should be retained indefinitely, usually with bonded retainers.

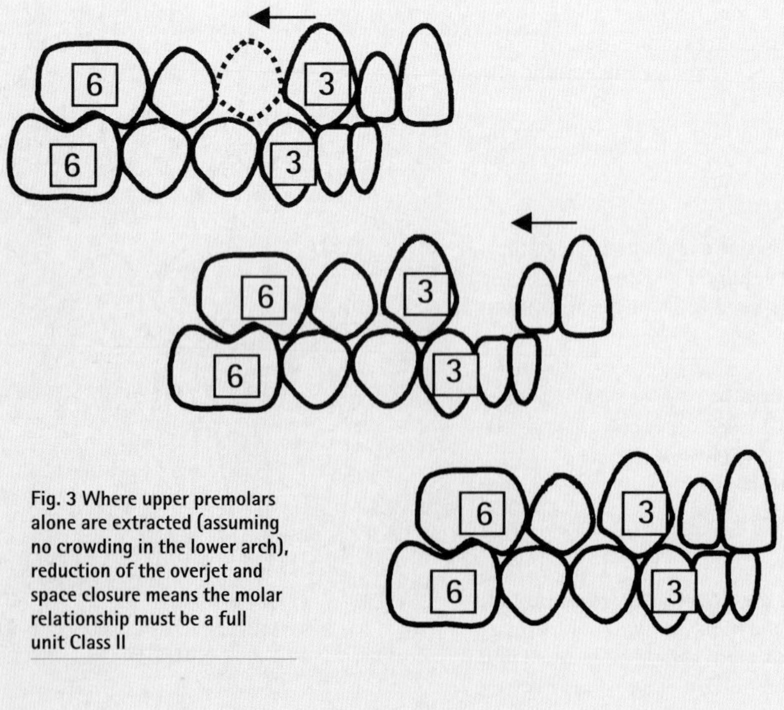

TREATMENT PLAN
The treatment plan should be considered as follows:

- Oral health
- Lower arch
- Upper arch
- Buccal occlusion
- Choose the appliance

Oral health
Tooth brushing and diet advice must be given and written in the notes. Daily fluoride rinses are also recommended. Caries must be treated and periodontal problems appropriately addressed.

Lower arch
Plan the lower arch first. The size and form of the lower arch should generally be accepted. Excessive expansion in the buccal regions or proclination of the lower incisors is contra-indicated in most cases because the soft tissues will generally return the teeth to their original position.

The need for extractions depends on the degree of crowding. In some cases, slight proclination of the lower incisors and expansion in the lower premolar region is acceptable, although this should be kept to a minimum and in carefully planned cases. Generally this type of treatment is confined to the correction of mild crowding (less than 5 mm), cases where incisors have been retroclined by a digit habit or trapped in the vault of the palate, or during development of Class II Division 2 malocclusions especially

Fig. 3 Where upper premolars alone are extracted (assuming no crowding in the lower arch), reduction of the overjet and space closure means the molar relationship must be a full unit Class II

where there is a deep bite. Any case where the overbite is excessive must be very carefully assessed before extraction decisions are made.

As the degree of crowding increases from 5–10 mm the need for extractions increases and with more than 10 mm of crowding extractions are nearly always required. If spontaneous alignment or removable appliances are to be used, first premolars are usually the extraction of choice because they are near to the site of crowding, allow the canines to upright and produce the best contact point relationship. If other teeth are to be extracted then generally fixed appliances will be required. Crowding tends to worsen with age and is thought to be related to facial growth which continues at least until the fifth decade.

Upper arch

Plan the upper arch around the lower. If extractions are undertaken in the lower arch these should generally be matched by extractions in the upper. If no extractions are carried out in the lower arch the space for upper arch alignment may come from either distal movement of the upper buccal segments or, extraction of upper premolars. The choice depends on the space requirements and the buccal occlusion. As the degree of crowding and overjet increase, then the space requirements will also increase and it is more likely that extractions as opposed to distal movement, will be indicated.

Determine whether the teeth are favourably positioned for spontaneous alignment. If appliances are needed can removable or fixed appliances accomplish the tooth movements?

Plan the buccal occlusion

Consider whether this needs to be corrected and if so how. If headgear is to be used, should it be used in conjunction with a removable or a fixed appliance? If the lower arch is crowded, space may be created by the removal of two lower premolars. This is then matched by upper premolar extractions and the molar relationship must be Class I at the end of treatment to allow the arches to fit together (Fig. 2).

However if the lower arch is well aligned, space to align the upper arch can be created by either upper premolar extractions or by distal movement of the upper buccal segments. The choice depends on how much space is required and what the molar relationship is at the start of treatment. Generally the more Class II the molars are the more likely one will opt for premolar extraction rather than distal movement. Moving molars more than 3–4 mm distally is

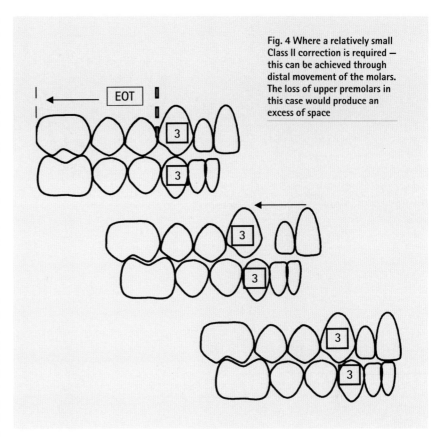

Fig. 4 Where a relatively small Class II correction is required — this can be achieved through distal movement of the molars. The loss of upper premolars in this case would produce an excess of space

possible but becomes increasingly demanding on patient co-operation. In circumstances where the space requirements are large, upper premolar extraction reduces the treatment time and increases patient compliance. Figure 3 shows the sequence of events when upper premolar extraction alone is undertaken as an aid to overjet reduction.

The nearer to Class I the initial buccal occlusion is, the more likely it will be that distal movement is appropriate. Therefore, space requirements that involve less than half a unit Class II correction can be accomplished by distal movement of the molars in a relatively short time with more chance of good patient co-operation (Fig. 4). Extracting upper premolars in these cases produces an excess of space and may increase the treatment time.

Choose the appliance

Once the need for extractions has been considered the appropriate appliance should be selected. This can involve allowing some spontaneous alignment to occur, using removable, fixed or functional appliances with the addition of extraoral traction or anchorage. Appliance choices are covered in the next section.

IN BRIEF

- The correct appliance choice is essential for optimum treatment outcome
- Removable appliances have an important but limited role in contemporary orthodontics
- Fixed appliances are usually the appliance of choice
- Functional appliances are helpful in difficult cases but may not have an effect on facial growth
- Extra-oral devices include headgear, face-masks and chin-caps

Appliance choices

D. Roberts-Harry and J. Sandy

There are bewildering array of different orthodontic appliances. However, they fall into four main categories of removable, fixed, functional and extra-oral devices. The appliance has to be selected with care and used correctly as inappropriate use can make the malocclusion worse. Removable appliances are only capable of very simple movements whereas fixed appliances are sophisticated devices, which can precisely position the teeth. Functional appliances are useful in difficult cases and are primarily used for Class II Division I malocciusions. Extra-oral devices are used to re-enforce anchorage and can be an aid in both opening and closing spaces.

There are four main types of types of appliance that can be used for orthodontic treatment. These are removable, fixed, functional and extra oral devices.

REMOVABLE APPLIANCES

In general these are only capable of simple tooth movement, such as tipping teeth. Bodily movement is very difficult to achieve with any degree of consistency and precise tooth detailing and multiple tooth movements are rarely satisfactory. These appliances have received bad press over the past few years because studies have shown that the treatment outcomes achieved can often be poor.[1,2] In these studies as many as 50% of cases treated with removable appliances were either not improved or worse than at the start of treatment. When faced with evidence such as this, one might be justified in discarding removable appliances completely. However, provided they are used in properly selected cases they still can be very useful devices and the treatment outcome can be satisfactory.[3] In general, removable appliances are only recommended for the following:

- Thumb deterrent
- Tipping teeth
- Block movements
- Overbite reduction
- Space maintenance
- Retention

Thumb deterrent

Digit sucking habits which persist into the teenage years can sometimes be hard to break and may result in either a posterior buccal cross bite or an anterior open bite with proclination of the upper and retroclination of the lower incisors. In general, if the habit stops before facial growth is complete then the anterior open bite usually resolves spontaneously and the overjet returns to normal.[4]

Figs. 1a–c show a case with an anterior open bite associated with an avid digit sucking habit. A simple upper removable appliance was used successfully to stop the habit. The appliance simply makes the habit feel less of a comfort and acts as a reminder to the patient that they should stop sucking the thumb. Complex appliances with bars or tongue cribs are rarely needed. In this patient once the habit had stopped the open bite closed down on its own without the need for further orthodontic treatment.

Tipping

One of the major uses of removable appliances is to move one incisor over the bite as shown in Figs 2a–d. A simple upper removable appliance utilized a 'T' spring constructed from 0.5 mm wire activated 1–2 mm which delivered a force of about 30 g to the tooth. After only a few weeks the cross bite was corrected without the need for complex treatment. Note the anterior

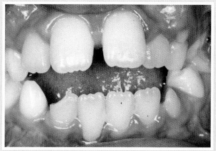

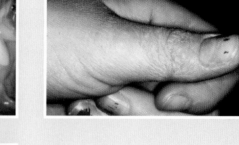

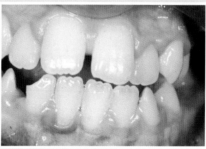

Fig. 1a–c A 9 year-old patient with an anterior open bite caused by a thumb sucking habit. Note the wear on the thumb as a result of this. She was fitted with a simple upper removable appliance and gently encouraged to stop the habit. She did so successfully and the open bite closed down spontaneously in 6 months

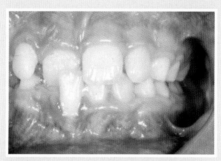

Fig. 2a an anterior cross bite involving the upper left and lower left central incisors

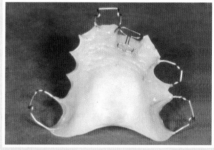

Fig. 2b An upper removable appliance with Adams cribs for retention made from 0.7 mm wire on the first permanent molars and the upper left central incisor. A 'T' spring made from 0.5 mm wire is used to push the tooth over the bite. The anterior retention is to prevent the front of the appliance being displaced as the spring is activated

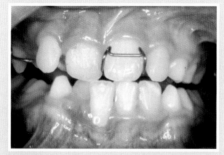

Fig. 2c The appliance in place. The T spring is activated 1–2 mm every 4 weeks

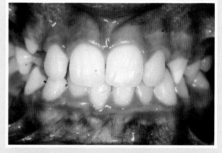

Fig. 2d The completed case. Active treatment took 12 weeks

retaining clasp that prevents the appliance from displacing downwards when the spring is activated.

If teeth are to be pushed over the bite with removable appliances, a stable result is more likely to be achieved if the tooth is retroclined in the first instance, the overbite is deep and there is an anterior mandibular displacement associated with a premature contact. Tipping teeth tends to reduce the overbite because the tip of the tooth moves along the arc of a circle as shown in Figure 3a. Excessive tipping may also make the tooth too horizontal which can be not only aesthetically unacceptable but may also

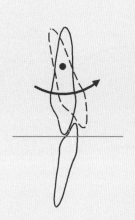

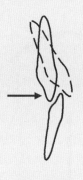

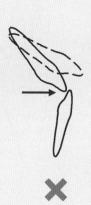

Fig. 3a The effect of tipping anterior teeth on the overbite. As the teeth move around a centre of rotation the incisal tip moves along the arc of a circle. By the laws of geometry, as the tooth is proclined the overbite reduces once it moves past the vertical

Fig. 3b Excessive tipping not only reduces the overbite but also makes the axial inclination of the teeth too horizontal. In these situations stability is reduced, the appearance is poor and the tooth may suffer from unwanted non-axial loading

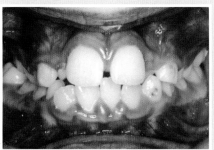

Fig. 4a Both the upper lateral incisors are in cross bite

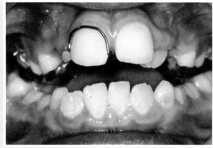

Fig. 4b An upper removable appliance was used to tip the laterals over the bite

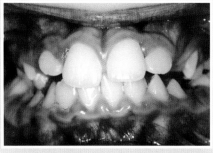

Fig. 4c The cross bites have been corrected. Note the reduction in the overbite

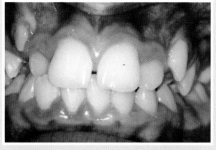

Fig. 4d 6 months later the upper right lateral has relapsed into cross bite due to the reduced overbite

result in excessive non-axial loading of the tooth as illustrated in Figure 3b.

Overbite reduction when teeth are over proclined is illustrated in Figures 4a–d. In this case both the upper lateral incisors were pushed over the bite with an upper removable appliance. The cross bite was corrected but note the reduction in overbite on the lateral incisors. Six months after completion of treatment the upper right lateral had relapsed back into cross bite.

Block movements

If a cross bite involves a number of teeth, for example, a unilateral buccal cross bite, removable appliances can be used to correct this. The sequence of events is shown in Figures 5a–f. Adams cribs are generally placed on the first premolars and the first permanent molars and a midline expansion screw is incorporated into the base plate. This midline screw is opened 0.25 mm (one quarter turn) twice a week until the cross bite is slightly overcorrected. Posterior buccal capping can also be used to disengage the bite and prevent concomitant expansion of the lower arch. Once the cross bite is corrected the buccal capping can be removed and the appliance used as a retainer to allow the buccal occlusion to settle in. Occasionally two appliances will be needed if a considerable amount of expansion is needed.

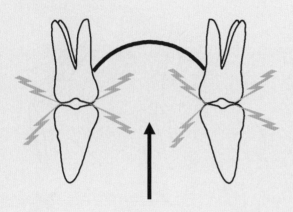

Fig. 5a Narrowness of the upper arch can produce a traumatic bite

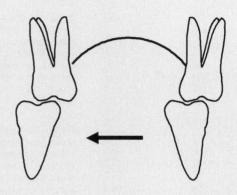

Fig. 5b To avoid painful cuspal contact the patient may move the mandible to one side producing a mandibular deviation and a cross bite

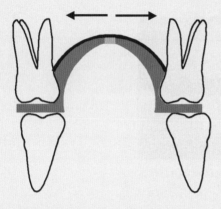

Fig. 5c An upper removable appliance with a mid line expansion screw can be used to correct the cross bite. The screw is opened one-quarter turn twice a week by the patient

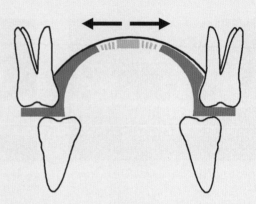

Fig. 5d The corrected cross bite. The treatment time varies with the amount of expansion needed but usually takes about twelve weeks

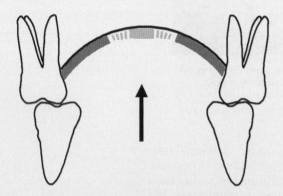

Fig. 5e Once active treatment is completed the appliance can be worn as a retainer. The posterior capping can be reduced to allow inter digitation of the buccal teeth thus helping to prevent any relapse

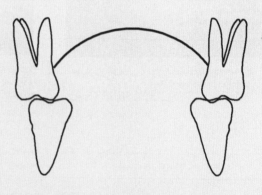

Fig. 5f The completed case

Overbite reduction

Removable appliances are very effective in correcting a deep overbite, especially in a growing patient. An upper removable appliance with an anterior bite plane is used which disengages the molars by 2–3 mm whilst at the same time establishing lower incisor contact with the bite plane (Fig. 6). Eruption of the posterior teeth produces a reduction in the overbite. It is essential that the inter-incisor angle is corrected at the completion of treatment so that an occlusal stop between the upper and lower incisors is produced preventing re-eruption of the incisors and a relapse of the overbite. Bite planes are usually used in conjunction with fixed appliances to help the overbite reduction (Figures 7a–d) or can be used as an aid to restoration of the anterior teeth. Figures 8a–d show a patient with a deep bite who had marked enamel erosion. Porcelain crowns were to be placed on the anterior teeth to restore them, but the deep bite made this technically difficult. The overbite

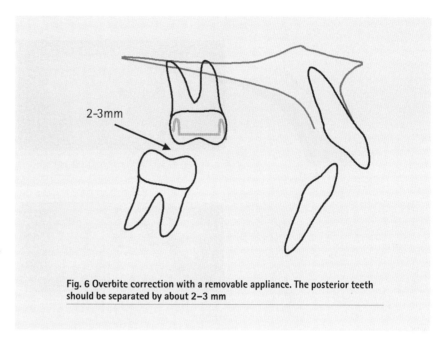

Fig. 6 Overbite correction with a removable appliance. The posterior teeth should be separated by about 2–3 mm

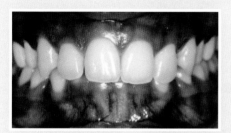

Fig. 7a A case with a deep bite and retroclined upper incisors

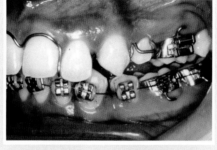

Fig. 7b An upper removable appliance is used to help the overbite reduction whilst palatal springs simultaneously move the first permanent molars distally

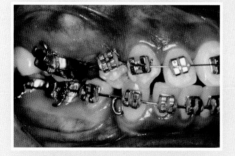

Fig. 7c Once the overbite is fully reduced the upper fixed appliance can be placed

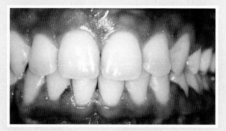

Fig. 7d The completed case with good overbite reduction

was therefore reduced with a bite plane to make room for the crowns.

Space maintenance

Space maintainers are rarely indicated in orthodontic treatment but occasionally can be used, particularly if the upper canine is buccally crowded. Whilst the extraction of the first premolars will often create space for the canines, there is a danger that the space will close before the canine erupts as the buccal teeth drift mesially. Figsures 9a–e illustrate such a case where the

fitting of a space maintainer proved useful. The appliance was fitted just prior to the emergence of the permanent canines. The four first premolars were then extracted and the appliance left in position until the canines erupted. This took about 6 months and saved a considerable amount of extra treatment for the patient by allowing spontaneous alignment of the canines.

Retention

Many orthodontists use various types of removable appliances to act as retainers, usually at the

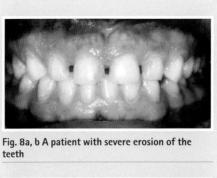

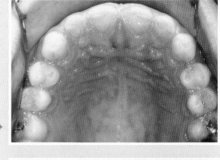

Fig. 8a, b A patient with severe erosion of the teeth

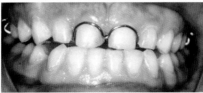

Fig. 8c A bite plane was used to reduce the overbite

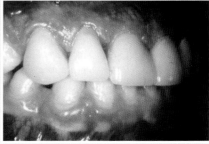

Fig. 8d Strip crowns were placed on the incisors once the overbite was reduced

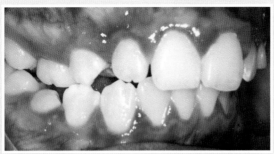

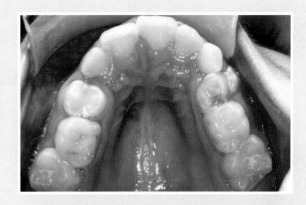

Fig. 9a, b A case with severe upper arch crowding. The upper permanent canines were unerupted, buccally positioned and very short of space

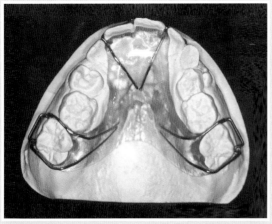

Fig. 9c An upper removable space maintainer. Adam cribs have been placed on the first permanent molars and a Southend clasp on the upper central incisors

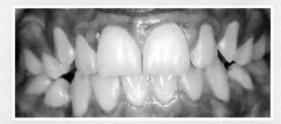

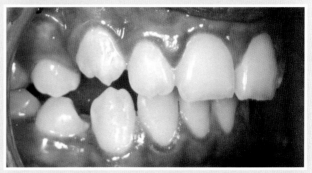

Fig. 9d,e The first premolars have been extracted and the upper canines are erupting into a good position

completion of fixed appliance treatment. Removable retainers are usually held in position with Adams Cribs on the first permanent molars with a labial bow and possible acrylic coverage of the anterior teeth (Fig. 10).

FIXED APPLIANCES

These appliances are attached to the crowns of teeth and allow correction of rotations, bodily movements of teeth and alignment of ectopic teeth. They have increased in sophistication enormously over the past 10–15 years and together with advancements in arch wire technology are capable of producing a very high level of treatment result. Simultaneous multiple

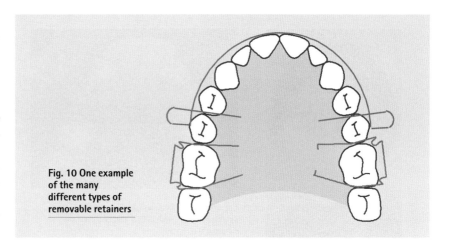

Fig. 10 One example of the many different types of removable retainers

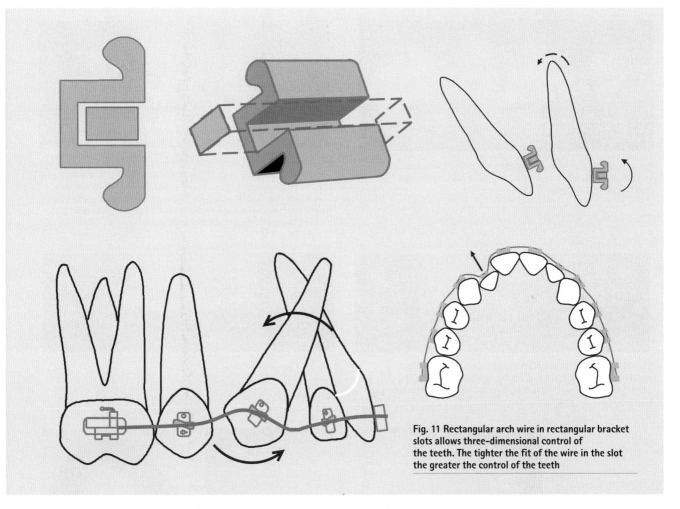

Fig. 11 Rectangular arch wire in rectangular bracket slots allows three-dimensional control of the teeth. The tighter the fit of the wire in the slot the greater the control of the teeth

tooth movements can be achieved, invariably creating a better treatment outcome than can be achieved with removable appliances. Although there are a variety of fixed appliances available they all operate in a similar way producing a fixed point of attachment to control the position of the teeth. Brackets are attached to the teeth and wires (arch wires) are placed in the bracket slots to move the teeth. The closer the fit of rectangular arch wires in a rectangular slot on the bracket the greater the control of the teeth (Fig 11). As treatment progresses, thicker rectangular wires are used to fully control the teeth in three dimensions. Fixed appliances are the appliances of choice for most orthodontic treat-

ment because the results are far more predictable and of a higher standard achieved than by other means. However, they are relatively complex appliances to use and further training in these devices is essential. An example of a case treated with fixed appliances is shown in Figure 12a–j. The anchorage requirements for the bodily movement of teeth are considerably greater than for tipping movements (Fig. 13).

FUNCTIONAL APPLIANCES

These are powerful appliances capable of impressive changes in the position of the teeth. They are generally used for Class II Division I malocclusions although they can be used for the

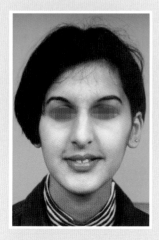

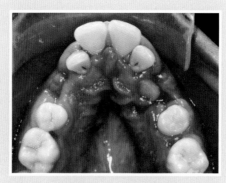

Fig. 12c Upper first and lower second premolars were extracted and the canines surgically exposed

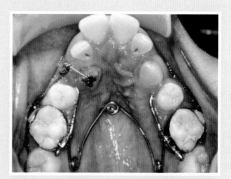

Fig. 12d A tri–helix was used to expand the upper arch and a sectional fixed appliance used to pull the canine into the line of the arch

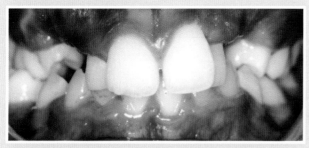

Fig. 12a, b Pre treatment photographs of a patient with palatally impacted canine, a buccal cross bite, an increased overjet and crowding in both arches

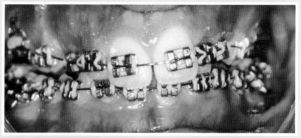

Fig. 12e Full fixed appliances were then used to reduce the over bite and overjet, move the apex of the canine into the line of the arch and correct all the other features of the malocclusion. The initial arch wire was a very thin flexible wire. If a thick wire is used at this stage excess force will be applied to the teeth that can produce root damage and be very painful for the patient

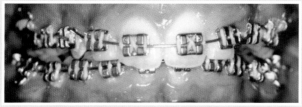

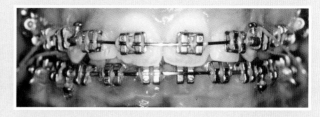

Figs 12f,g Once initial alignment of the teeth is produced progressively thicker, stiffer wires are employed. Because these fit the bracket slot more closely they control tooth position more precisely than the thinner aligning wires

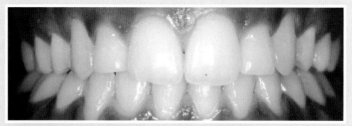

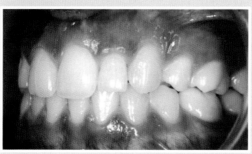

Fig. 12h,i The completed case. The canine is fully aligned and the overjet reduced without any unwanted tipping of the teeth

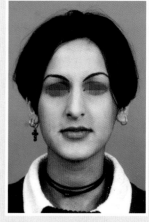

Fig. 12j Appropriate extractions and treatment mechanics have not been detrimental to the facial appearance

correction of Class II Division II and Class III malocclusions on occasion. They are either removable from the mouth or fixed to the teeth, and work by stimulating the muscles of mastication and soft tissues of the face. This produces a distalising force on the upper dentition and an anterior force on the lower. Whilst they are capable of substantial tooth movement, like all removable appliances they are not capable of precise tooth positioning and cannot deal effectively with rotations or bodily tooth movement.

There is some controversy as to the precise mode of action of functional appliances. Some clinicians feel they have an effect on this facial skeleton, promoting growth of the mandible and/or maxilla. Others feel that the effects are mainly dento-alveolar and that the results achieved are accomplished by tipping the upper and lower teeth. Unfortunately many of the studies relating to functional appliance treatment have been poorly constructed and their conclusions should be treated with caution. A large-scale, prospective, randomized clinical trial currently being undertaken in United Kingdom strongly suggests that 98% of the occlusal

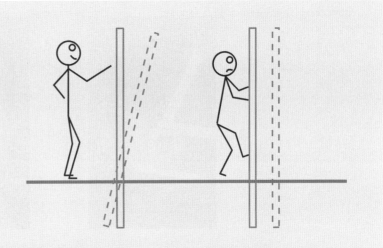

Fig. 13 Bodily movement of the teeth requires a greater degree of force than tipping movements

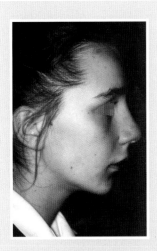

Fig. 14a,b Pre-treatment photographs of a 12-year-old girl with an increased overjet and a class II skeletal pattern associated with a retrognathic mandible

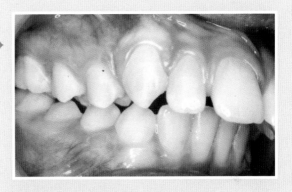

Fig. 14c A functional appliance was used to correct the saggital relationship

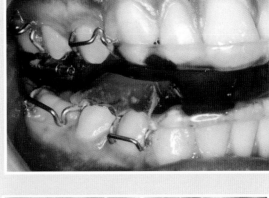

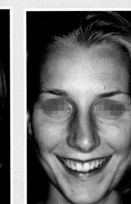

Fig. 14e,f The facial appearance following treatment

Fig. 14d The final result after detailing of the occlusion with fixed appliances

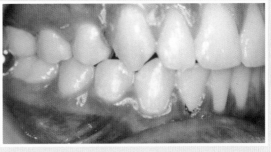

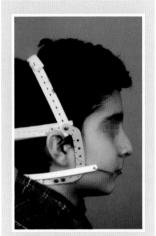

Fig. 15 Extra-oral traction applied via an Interlandii headgear

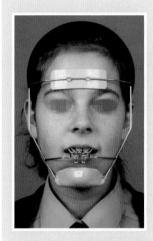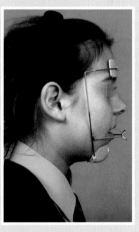

Fig. 16a,b A facemask or reverse headgear

correction is by tipping of the teeth with an almost negligible effect on the skeletal pattern.[5] Nevertheless, dramatic occlusal changes are possible with these appliances and they can aid the correction of some quite severe malocclusions. Figures 14a–f show a case treated with a functional appliance that had a marked effect not only on the occlusion but also on the patient's facial appearance.

EXTRA-ORAL DEVICES

These are headgear devices, chin caps and face masks, which are used to provide an external source of anchorage or traction for teeth in one or both arches. The commonest type is headgear for the distal movement of the buccal teeth. A metal face bow is attached to either a removable or a fixed appliance inside the mouth and elastic traction applied to it. As well as force being applied distally to either the maxilla or the mandible it can be applied mesially via a facemask. This is typically used in Class III cases to correct an ante-rior cross bite or in cases where the buccal segments are being moved forwards to close spaces in the arches. Examples of extra oral traction devices are shown in Figures 15, 16a and b. Chin caps have been used to try and restrain mandibular growth in Class III malocclusions. However, the evidence from the literature suggests that they are not terribly effective and their use has declined in recent years.

1. Richmond S, Shaw W C, O'Brien K D et al. The development of the Par index (Peer Assessment Rating): reliability and validity. Eur J Orthod 1992; **14:** 125-139.
2. Richmond S, Shaw W C, Roberts C T, Andrews M. The PAR index (Peer Assessment rating): methods to determine the outcome of orthodontic treatment in terms of improvements and standards. Eur J Orthod 1992; **14:** 180-187.
3. Kerr W J S, Buchanan I B, McColl J H. The use of the PAR index in assessing the effectiveness of removable orthodontic appliances. Br J Orthod 1993; **20:** 351-357.
4. Leighton B C. The early signs of malocclusion. Trans Europ Orthod Soc 1969; 353-368.
5. O'Brien K, Wright J, Conboy F et al. Effectiveness of treatment for Class II malocclusion with the Herbst or twin-block appliances: a randomized, controlled trial. Am J Orthod Dentofacial Orthop 2003; **124:** 128-137.

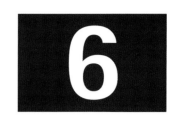
IN BRIEF

- Before any active orthodontic treatment is considered it is essential that the oral hygiene is of a high standard and that all carious leions have been dealt with
- Arch wires, headgears and brackets themselves may cause significant damage either during an active phase of treatment or during debonding. Much care needs to be taken when instructing patients about their role in orthodontic treatment
- The aim of this section is to outline potential risks in orthodontic treatment and to give examples. There are also a number of illustrations to help highlight these points

Risks in orthodontic treatment

H. Travess*, D. Roberts-Harry and J. Sandy

Orthodontics has the potential to cause significant damage to hard and soft tissues. The most important aspect of orthodontic care is to have an extremely high standard of oral hygiene before and during orthodontic treatment. It is also essential that any carious lesions are dealt with before any active treatment starts. Root resorption is a common complication during orthodontic treatment but there is some evidence that once appliances are removed this resorption stops. Some of the risk pointers for root resorption are summarised. Soft tissue damage includes that caused by archwires but also the more harrowing potential for headgears to cause damage to eyes. It is essential that adequate safety measures are included with this type of treatment.

*Senior Specialist Registrar, Orthodontic Department, Leeds Dental Institute, Clarendon Way, Leeds LS2 9LU

If orthodontic treatment is to be of benefit to a patient, the advantages it offers should outweigh any possible damage it may cause.[1] It is important to assess the risks of treatment as well as the potential gain and balance these aspects of treatment before deciding to treat a malocclusion. The psychological trauma of having orthodontic treatment, or indeed not having treatment should not be overlooked and is an important consideration in treatment planning. Patient selection plays a vital role in minimising risks of treatment and the clinician should be vigilant in assessing every aspect of the patient and their malocclusion. However, clinically there are a number of areas of concern for risk management. These are discussed in detail under the broad categories of intra-oral, extra-oral and systemic risks.

INTRA–ORAL RISKS

Enamel demineralisation/caries

Enamel demineralisation, usually on smooth surfaces, is unfortunately a common complication in orthodontics, figures range from 2–96% of orthodontic patients (Fig.1).[2] This large variation probably arises as a result of the variety of methods used to assess and score the presence of decalcification. There is also inconsistency on whether idiopathic lucencies are included or excluded in the study design.[3] The teeth most commonly affected are maxillary lateral incisors, maxillary canines and mandibular premolars.[4] However, any tooth in the mouth can be affected, and often a number of anterior teeth show decal-

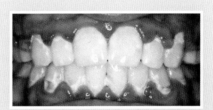

Fig. 1 Decalcification on labial surfaces of numerous teeth

cification. Whilst the demineralised surface remains intact, there is a possibility of remineralisation and reversal of the lesion. In severe cases, frank cavitation is seen which requires restorative intervention (Figs. 2 and 3).

Gorelick et al.[5] in a study on white spot formation in children treated with fixed appliances, found that half of their patients had at least one white spot after treatment, most commonly on maxillary lateral incisors. The length of treatment did not affect the incidence or number of white spot formations, although O'Reilly and Featherstone[6] and Oggard et al.[7] found that demineralisation can occur rapidly, within the first month of fixed appliance treatment. This has obvious aesthetic implications and highlights the need for caries rate assessment at the beginning of treatment. Interestingly, Gorelick et al.[5] found no incidence of white spot formation associated with lingual bonded retainers, which would suggest salivary buffering capacity, and flow rate have a role in protection against acid attack.

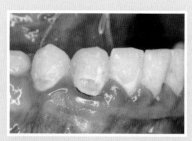
Fig. 2 Cavitation at the gingival margin of the lower right canine and first premolar requiring restoration

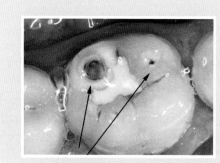
Fig. 3 Obvious caries in the disto-occlusal aspect of a lower molar

or by adjunct fluoride mouthwash (0.05% sodium fluoride daily rinse or 0.2% sodium fluoride weekly rinse), can be helpful in remineralising the lesion and reducing the unsightliness of the decalcification.[10] Acid/pumice micro abrasion has also been advocated to improve the aesthetics of stabilised lesions.[11,12] This procedure should be delayed at least 3 months following debond to allow for spontaneous improvement of the lesions and remineralisation with fluoride applications.[13] Persistent lucencies should be abraded with 18% hydrochloric acid in fine pumice under rubber dam in bursts of 30 seconds for a maximum of 10 times. After the last application the tooth is washed well and a fluoride varnish applied.[11]

Enamel trauma

When placing appliances careless use of a band seater can result in enamel fracture. Care is required when large restorations are present since these can result in fracture of unsupported cusps.[14] Debonding can also result in enamel fracture, both with metal and ceramic brackets (Fig. 4).[15,16] Care must always be taken to remove brackets and residual bonding agents appropriately to minimise the risk of enamel fracture. The use of debonding burs has the potential to remove enamel, especially in air turbine fast handpieces. Care and attention is needed when adhesives are removed.

Enamel wear

Wear of enamel against both metal and ceramic brackets (abrasion) may occur. It is common on upper canine tips during retraction as the cusp tip hits the lower canine brackets (Fig. 5). It may also be seen on the incisal edges of upper anterior teeth where ceramic brackets are placed on lower incisors.[17] Ceramic brackets are very abrasive and therefore contraindicated for the lower anterior teeth where there is any possibility of the brackets occluding with the upper teeth, bearing in mind that the overbite may

- **Good oral hygiene is essential for successful orthodontic treatment**
- **Daily fluoride rinses may prevent and reduce decalcifications**
- **Care is needed when debracketing as there is the potential for enamel damage especially with ceramic brackets**

The dominant hand may also influence the area of decalcification as brushing is more difficult on the side of the dominant hand. Whilst good oral hygiene is vital, dietary control of sugar intake is also needed in order to minimise the risk of decalcification. Fluoride mouthwashes used throughout treatment can prevent white spot formation[8] surprisingly, compliance with this is low (13%). Other fluoride release mechanisms include fluoride releasing bonding agents, elastic ligatures containing fluoride, and depot devices on upper molar bands.[9]

Preventive measures to minimise damage include patient selection, vigorous oral hygiene measures and dietary education. Reinforcement of oral hygiene and dietary education should be performed at each visit. Positive reinforcement even where oral hygiene is satisfactory will encourage the patient further. Inspection of the labial surfaces of the teeth at each adjustment appointment will identify cases that require more intervention and advice. It is important when examining the teeth that they are plaque-free otherwise early demineralisation may be missed. This can be done by instructing the patient to clean their teeth in the surgery with or without the wires in place, or by professional prophylaxis. The use of auxillaries such as dental health educators and hygienists is highly desirable. Removal of the appliance in cases with extreme demineralisation or poor hygiene is the last resort, but should not be discounted by the clinician.

Where demineralisation is present post treatment, fluoride application either via toothpaste,

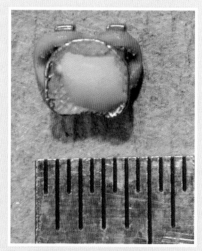
Fig. 4 Enamel fracture at debond

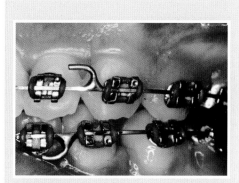

Fig. 5 Upper canine tip showing abrasion from the lower canine metal bracket

increase in the early stages of treatment. Any enamel erosion must be recorded prior to treatment commencing and appropriate dietary advice given to minimise further tooth substance loss. Carbonated drinks and pure juices are the commonest causes of erosion and should be avoided in patients with fixed appliances.

Pulpal reactions
Some degree of pulpitis is expected with orthodontic tooth movement which is usually reversible or transient. Rarely it leads to loss of vitality, but there may be an increase in pulpitis in previously traumatised teeth with fixed appliances. Light forces are advocated with traumatised teeth as well as baseline monitoring of vitality which should be repeated three monthly.[18] Transient pulpitis may also be seen with electrothermal debonding of ceramic brackets[19] and composite removal at debond.[20]

Root resorption
Some degree of external root resorption is inevitably associated with fixed appliance treatment, although the extent is unpredictable.[21] Resorption may occur on the apical and lateral surface of the roots, but radiographs only show apical resorption to a certain degree. Many cases will not show any clinically significant resorption but, microscopic changes are likely to have occurred on surfaces which are not visualised with routine radiographs. Resorption however, rarely compromises the longevity of the teeth.[22] Vertical loss of bone through periodontal disease creates a far greater loss of attachment and support than it's equivalent loss around the apex of a tooth.

The mechanism of tooth resorption is unclear. Theories include excessive force and hyalinisation of the periodontal ligament resulting in excessive cementoclast and osteoclast activity. What is clear are the risk factors which are associated with cases with severe resorption. These can be summarised:

- Blunt and pipette shaped roots show a greater amount of resorption than other root forms.

- Short roots are more at risk of resorption than average length roots.
- Teeth previously traumatised, have an increased risk of further resorption.
- Non vital teeth and root treated teeth have an increased risk of resorption.
- Heavy forces are associated with resorption, as well as the use of rectangular wires, Class II traction, the distance a tooth is moved and the type of tooth movement undertaken.
- Combined orthodontic and orthognathic procedures.

Treatment of ectopic canines may induce resorption of the adjacent teeth because of the length of treatment time and the distance the canine is moved. Tooth intrusion is also associated with increased risk as well as movement of root apices against cortical bone. Above the age of 11 years the risk of resorption with treatment seems to increase. Adults have shorter roots at the outset and the potential for resorption is increased.

Opinion is divided on whether treatment length is associated with increased resorption. Some find no correlation with treatment time, whereas others find that there is increased resorption with increased treatment time. In a few patients systemic causes may contribute for example hyperthyroidism, but for the most part no underlying cause is isolated other than individual susceptibility. Familial risk is also known.

A wide range in the degree of resorption is seen, highlighting the role of individual susceptibility over and above the risk factors identified. Research is still required in this area to identify the mechanisms of resorption, trigger factors and reparative mechanisms if treatment modalities are to be modified in the future to minimise root damage. Currently, no case is immune from the risk of root resorption, to some degree, and patients should be warned at the outset of treatment that such a risk exists. Recognition of specific risk factors, accurate radiographs and interpretation of radiographs at the outset of treatment are important if root resorption is to be minimised. Once resorption is recognised clinically during treatment, light forces must be used, root length monitored six monthly with radiographs and treatment aims reconsidered to maximise the longevity of the dentition. The use of thyroxine to minimise root resorption has been advocated by some authors, but this is not routinely used.[23, 24]

Periodontal tissues
Fixed appliances make oral hygiene difficult even for the most motivated patients, and almost all patients experience some gingival inflammation (Fig. 6). Resolution of inflammation usually occurs a few weeks after debond, bands cause more gingival inflammation than bonds, which is not surprising since the margins of bands are often seated subgingivally.

- Root resorption is inevitable with fixed appliance treatment
- On average 1–2 mm of apical root is lost during a course of orthodontic treatment
- Previously traumatised teeth have an increased risk of root resorption

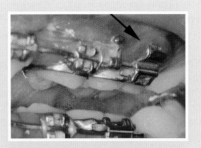

Fig. 6 Severe gingival inflammation during fixed appliance treatment. Note the inflammation covers the headgear tube and hook on the upper molar band

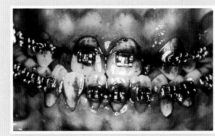

Fig. 7 Disclosing solution highlighting the areas of poor oral hygiene in a patient

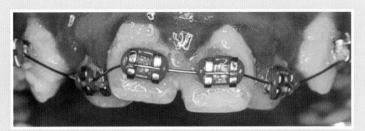

Fig. 8 Chronic lack of oral hygiene showing accumulation of plaque gingivally and around the brackets

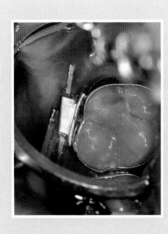

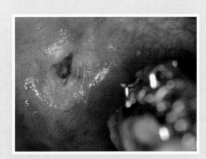

Fig. 9 Trauma to the cheek from an unusally long distal length of archwire resulting in an ulcer

For the most part, the literature suggests that orthodontic treatment does not affect the periodontal status of patients over the long term. Patients with pre-existing periodontal disease require special attention, but bone loss during treatment does not seem to be related to previous bone loss. The need for excellent oral hygiene during treatment must be emphasised in patients with existing periodontal disease. The use of bonds rather than bands on molars and premolars may be more appropriate to eliminate unwanted stagnation areas. Plaque retention is increased with fixed appliances and plaque composition may also be altered. There is an increase in anaerobic organisms and a reduction in facultative anaerobes around bands, which are therefore periopathogenic.[25]

Oral hygiene instruction is essential in all cases of orthodontic treatment, and the use of adjuncts such as electric toothbrushes, interproximal brushes, chlorhexidine mouthwashes, fluoride mouthwashes and regular professional cleaning must be emphasised. However, patient motivation and dexterity are paramount in the success of hygiene, and there will always be cases where oral hygiene is unsatisfactory from the outset. This should be carefully considered when advising a patient to have treatment. Experience shows those patients who are unable to maintain a healthy oral environment in the absence of fixed orthodontics will fail spectacularly with braces in place. Benefit must therefore significantly outweigh the risk of carrying out treatment in such patients (Figs. 7 and 8).

Allergy
Allergy to orthodontic components intraorally is exceedingly rare, however, there have been studies on the nickel release and corrosion of metals with fixed appliances. Gjerdet et al.[26] found a significant release of nickel and iron into the saliva of patients just after placement of fixed appliances. However, no significant difference was found in nickel or iron concentrations between controls and subjects where the appliances had been in place for a number of weeks. The clinical significance of nickel release is as yet unclear, but should be considered in nickel sensitive patients. There are a few cases with severe latex allergies who may be affected by elastomerics or operators gloves.

Trauma
Laceration to the gingivae, and mucosa seen as areas of ulceration or hyperplasia, often occur during treatment or between treatment sessions from the archwire (Fig. 9) and bonds, especially where long unsupported stretches of wire rest against the lips. The use of dental wax over the bracket may help to reduce trauma and discomfort, (Fig. 10) as may rubber bumper sleeving on the unsupported archwire (Fig. 11).

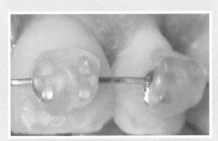

Fig. 10 Dental wax placed over a bracket can ease the pain of ulceration in the lip and mucosa

EXTRA-ORAL RISKS

Allergy

Allergy to nickel is more common in extra-oral settings, most usually the headgear face bow or head strap. Over 1% of patients have some form of contact dermatitis to zips and buttons/studs on clothing. Of these patients, 3% claim to have experienced a similar rash with orthodontic appliances (Fig. 12). The use of sticking plaster over the area in contact with the skin is sufficient to relieve symptoms. Allergy to latex[27] and bonding materials has been reported although these are rare.

Trauma

Following a well publicised case of eye trauma in a patient wearing headgear[28] a number of safety headgear products have been designed and explicit guidelines are now available. These measures include safety bows (Figs 13 and 14), rigid neck straps (Fig. 15) and snap release products (Fig. 16) to prevent the bow from disengaging from the molar tubes or acting as a projectile. A survey among British orthodontists found a 4% incidence of facial injury with headgear. Of these injuries, 40% were extra-oral and 50% of these were in the mid face. Two patients were blind as a result of headgear trauma. Eye injury is uncommon, but a serious risk and all available methods of reducing the risk of penetrating eye injury must be used. Every headgear and Kloehn

bow must incorporate a safety feature. Failure to observe safety guidelines on the use of headgear is medico-legally indefensible.

Burns

Burns, either thermal or chemical are possible both intra- and extra-orally with inadvertent use of chemicals or instruments. Acid etch, electrothermal debonding instruments and sterilised instruments which have not cooled down all have the potential to burn and care should be taken in their use.

Tempromandibular dysfunction (TMD)

Much attention in the literature has been focused on the relationship between TMD and orthodontic treatment. Whilst TMD is common in the orthodontic aged population whether orthodontic treatment is carried out or not, there is no evidence to support the theory that orthodontic treatment causes TMD or cures it.[29] Pre-existence of TMD should be recorded, and the patient advised that treatment will not predictably improve their condition. Some patients may suffer with increased symptoms during treatment which must also be discussed at the beginning of treatment. Where patients experience symptoms during treatment, treatment should be directed at eliminating occlusal disharmony and joint noises whilst reassuring the patient. Standard

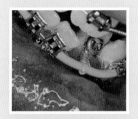

Fig. 11 Ulcer in a patient's lower lip from a long stretch of unsupported wire. Bumper sleeve has been placed along the wire to prevent further trauma

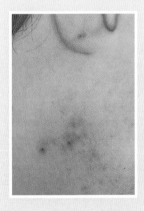

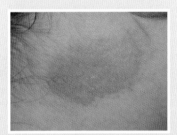

Fig. 12 Nickel allergy (contact dermatitis) in a headgear wearer

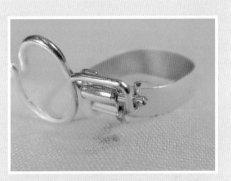

Fig. 13 Safety Kloehn bow showing recurved loops for smooth distal ends to prevent injury if the bow becomes disengaged

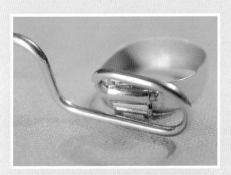

Fig. 14 Safety Kloehn bow with Nitom locking mechanism to prevent disengagement from the molar tube

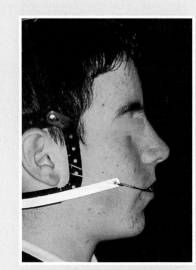

Fig. 15 Interlandi headgear with a rigid Masel safety strap to hold the Kloehn bow and prevent disengagement for the buccal tubes

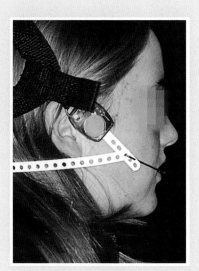

Fig. 16 Quick release headgear attachment. The breakaway design allows the bow to come out of the headgear tube, but is no longer under tension and therefore unable to act as a projectile

treatment regimes may also be indicated eg soft diet, jaw exercises. We have not reviewed this area in detail in this section as it is dealt with under facts and fantasy in the next, but an excellent overview of the relation between orthodontics and occlusal relation has recently been published.[30]

Profile damage

Extraction of premolars has been condemned by some with very little evidence, as altering the facial profile of the patient.[31] A large number of studies have shown that there is no significant difference in profiles treated by extraction or non extraction means. Boley *et al.*[32] found that neither orthodontists nor general dentists could distinguish between extraction and non extraction treatment by looking at profile alone. A recent review examined the effects of orthodontics on facial profie and concluded that it does not, although it highlights areas where planning is crucial.[33] It should be remembered that soft tissue changes occur naturally with age, regardless of orthodontic intervention. Proper diagnosis should take into account skeletal form, tooth position and soft tissue form to negate the possibility of any detrimental effect on profile by treatment mechanics.[34]

SYSTEMIC RISKS

Cross infection

Spread of infection between patients, between operator and patient and by a third party should be prevented by cross infection procedures throughout the surgery. Use of gloves, masks, sterilised instruments and 'clean' working areas are paramount. A medical history must be taken for every patient to determine risk factors,

although cross infection control should be of a standard to prevent cross contamination regardless of medical status.

Infective endocarditis

Patients at risk of endocarditis should be treated in consultation with their cardiologist and within the appropriate guidelines.[35,36] The patient must exhibit immaculate oral hygiene, antibiotic cover will be required for invasive procedures such as extractions, separation, band placement and band removal. It is recommended that bonded attachments are used on all teeth to negate the need for antibiotic cover for both separator and band placement, as well as removal. This also reduces the risk of unwanted plaque stagnation areas. Chlorhexidine mouthwash has been advocated prior to any treatment and in some cases daily to minimise bacterial loading.[36]

CONCLUSIONS

Clearly there are a number of sources of potential iatrogenic damage to the patient during orthodontic treatment. However, severe damage is rare. Severe malocclusions have more to benefit from treatment than less severe malocclusions, and motivation between such groups may vary. Individuals should be assessed for risk factors for all aspects of care. Lack of treatment can result in damage, physical or psychosocial. Discontinuation of treatment without full correction of the malocclusion, although a last resort, can leave the patient worse off than before treatment. Good clinical practice, careful patient selection and information on a patient's responsibility are essential to minimise tissue damage.

The authors are grateful to Francis Scriven , Thomas Hartridge and Ingrid Hosein for some of the figures and Jane Western who cheerfully typed this manuscript.

1. Shaw W C, O'Brien K D, Richmond S, Brook P. Quality control in orthodontics: risk/benefit considerations. *Br Dent J* 1991; **170:** 33-37.

2. Chang H S, Walsh L J, Freer T J. Enamel demineralisation during orthodontic treatment. Aetiology and prevention. *Aus Dent J* 1997; **42:** 322-327.

3. Mitchell L. Decalcification during orthodontic treatment with fixed appliances — An overview. *Br J Orthod* 1992 ; **19:** 199-205.

4. Geiger A M, Gorelick L, Gwinnett A J, Griswold P G. The effect of a fluoride program on white spot formation during orthodontic treatment. *Am J Orthod Dento Orthop* 1988; **93:** 29-37.

5. Gorelick L, Geiger A M, Gwinnett A J. Incidence of white spot formation after bonding and banding. *Am J Orthod* 1982; **81:** 93-98.

6. O'Reilly M, Featherstone J. Demineralisation and remineralisation around orthodontic appliances — an *in vivo* study. *Am J Orthod Dento Orthop* 1987; **92:** 33-40.

7. Öggard B, Rølla G, Arends J. Orthodontic appliances and enamel demineralisation. Part 1. Lesion development. *Am J Orthod Dento Orthop* 1988; **94:** 68-73.

8. Geiger A M, Gorelick L, Gwinnett A J, Griswold P G. Effect of a fluoride program on white spot formation during orthodontic treatment. *Am J Orthod Dento Orthop* 1988; **93:** 29-37.

9. Marini I, Pelliccioni G A, Vecchiet F, Alessandri Bonetti G, Checchi L. A retentive system for intra-oral fluoride release during orthodontic treatment. *Eur J Orthod* 1999; **21:** 695-701.

10. Featherstone J D B, Rodgers B E, Smith M W. Physiochemical requirements for rapid remineralisation of early carious lesions. *Caries Res* 1981; **15:** 221-235.

11. Welbury R R, Carter N E. The hydrochloric acid-pumice microabrasion technique in the treatment of post orthodontic decalcification. *Br J Orthod* 1993; **108:** 181-185.

12. Elkhazindar M M, Welbury R R. Enamel Microabrasion. *Dent Update* 2000; **27:** 194-196.

13. Artun J, Thylstrup A. Clinical and scanning electron microscopic study of surface changes of incipient caries lesions after debonding. *Scand J Dent Res* 1986; **94:** 193-201.

14. McGuinness N. Prevention in orthodontics — a review. *Dent Update* 1992; **19:** 168-175.

15. Meister R E. Comparison of enamel detachments after debonding between uniteck's dynalok bracket and a foil mesh bracket: a scanning electron microscope study. *Am J Orthod* 1985; **88:** 266 (abstract).

16. Jones M. Enamel loss on bond removal. *Br J Orthod* 1980; **7:** 39.

17. Swartz M L. Ceramic brackets. *J Clin Orthod* 1988; **22:** 82-88.

18. Atack N E. The orthodontic implications of traumatised upper anterior teeth. *Dent Update* 1999; **26:** 432-437.

19. Takla P M, Shivapuja P K. Pulpal response in electrothermal debonding. *Am J Orthod Dento Orthop* 1995; **108:** 623-629.

20. Zachrisson B U. Cause and prevention of injuries to teeth and supporting structures during orthodontic treatment. *Am J Orthod* 1976; **69:** 285-300.

21. Brezniak N, Wasserstein A. Root resorption after orthodontic treatment Part I Literature review. *Am J Orthod* 1993; **103:** 62-66.

22. Hendrix I, Carels C, Kuijpers-Jagtman A M, Van 'T Hof M. A radiographic study of posterior apical root resorption in orthodontic patients. *Am J Orthod Dento Orthop* 1994; **105:** 345-349.

23. Shirazi M, De Hpour A R, Jafari F. The effect of thyroid hormaone on orthodontic tooth movement in rats. *J Clin Paed Dent* 1999; **23:** 259-264.

24. Loberg E L, Engstrom C. Thyroid administration to reduce root resorption. *Angle Orthod* 1994; **64:** 395-399.

25. Diamanti-Kipioti A, Gusberti F A, Lang N P. Clinical microbiological effects of fixed orthodontic appliances. *J Clin Perio* 1987; **14:** 326-333.

26. Gjerdet N, Erichsen E S, Remlo H E, Evjen G. Nickel and iron in saliva of patients with fixed orthodontic appliances. *Acta Odont Scand* 1991; **49:** 73-78.

27. Natrass C, Ireland A J, Lovell C R. Latex allergy in an orthodontic patient and implications for clinical management. *Br J Oral Maxillofac Surg* 1999; **37:** 11-13.

28. Booth-Mason S, Birnie D. Penetrating eye injury from orthodontic headgear: a case report. *Eur J Orthod* 1988; **10:** 111-114.

29. Luther F. Orthodontics and the temperomandibular joint: where are we now? Part 1 Orthodontic treatment and temperomandibular disorders. *Angle Orthod* 1998; **68:** 295-304.

30. Davies S J, Gray R M J, Sandler P J, O'Brien K D. Orthodontics and occlusion. *Br Dent J* 2001; **191:** 539-549.

31. Rushing S E, Silberman S L, Meydrech E F, Tuncay O C. How dentists perceive the effect of orthodontic extraction on facial appearance. *J Am Dent Assoc* 1995; **126:** 769-772.

32. Boley J C, Pontier J P, Smith S, Fulbright M. Facial changes in extraction and non extraction patients. *Angle Orthod* 1998; **68:** 539-546.

33. DiBiase A T, Sandler P J. Does Orthodontics damage faces? *Dent Update* 2001; **28:** 98-104.

34. Ackerman J L, Proffit W R. Soft tissue limitations in orthodontics: treatment planning guidelines. *Angle Orthod* 1997; **67:** 327-336

35. Khurana M, Martin M V. Orthodontics and infective endocarditis. *Br J Orthod* 1999; **26:** 295-298.

36. Hobson R S, Clark J D. Management of the orthodontic patient at risk from infective endocarditis. *Br Dent J* 1995; **178:** 289-295.

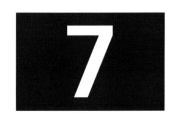

IN BRIEF

- There is no good evidence that orthodontics cures or causes temporomandibular joint dysfunction
- Extracting teeth does not inevitably result in an altered profile
- There is a need for better quality research in many of the controversial areas in orthodontics

Fact and fantasy in orthodontics

P. Williams*, D. Roberts-Harry and J. Sandy

Clinical research has previously lacked good methodology and much opinion was based on anecdote which is widely regarded as the weakest form of clinical evidence. There are few randomised control trials in orthodontics which support or refute areas of dogma. The number of randomised control trials is increasing significantly. There is currently however no good evidence that orthodontics causes or cures temporomandibular joint dysfunction, that appropriate extractions in orthodontics ruin patients' profiles, or that the orthodontist is able to significantly influence facial growth with appliances.

Orthodontics, like other fields of medicine and dentistry has its fair share of controversies. Some of these controversies have haunted the profession since its inception and some individuals may be reluctant to change their treatment philosophies in the light of new clinical evidence.

Orthodontics has evolved from many years of clinical experience, in which the opinions of respected individuals during the birth of the speciality have determined how orthodontics should be practised. A problem with this form of teaching is that it is based on anecdotal experience rather than sound scientific evidence. New research often highlights inadequacies in these fundamental teachings, eventually leading to a change in clinical practice. A trend is emerging towards evidence-based rather than opinion-based decisions as more and more structured research is published.

EVIDENCE-BASED DECISIONS

Evidence-based dentistry can be defined as: 'the conscientious, explicit, and judicious use of current best evidence in making decisions about the care of individual patients'.[1] The 'gold standard' is strong evidence from at least one published systematic review of multiple well-designed randomised controlled trails. Meta-analysis is a form of systematic review looking at all the relevant literature whether good, bad or indifferent and producing a single estimate of the clinical effectiveness. The advantage of meta-analysis is that it summarises the available evidence and because of its systematic nature it can be appraised rapidly and applied to patient care.[2]

There are various levels of evidence beneath the 'gold standard', of which the weakest is anecdotal evidence. In the field of orthodontics there are few well-designed randomised controlled trials which lend themselves to a systematic review. Currently there are two such reviews, namely the change of intercanine width following orthodontic treatment and the treatment of posterior crossbites.[3,4]

Recently, media attention has focused on views made by a small number of orthodontists and general dental practitioners on the adverse effects of conventional orthodontic treatment. Much of this has centred on the role of extracting teeth as part of orthodontic therapy to align teeth, retract protrusive incisors and to camouflage dentally any skeletal disharmonies between the mandible and the maxillae.

Summary of evidence-based dentistry
- Anecdotal evidence is the weakest form of evidence
- 'Gold standard' is a randomised controlled trial
- Orthodontics has little 'gold standard' evidence

ORTHODONTICS AND TEMPOROMANDIBULAR DYSFUNCTION

Relatively recently, orthodontists have been concerned about the possibility of a link between the orthodontic treatment they provide and temporomandibular dysfunction (TMD) which is a

*Specialist Registrar in Orthodontics, Division of Child Dental Health, University of Bristol Dental School, Lower Maudlin Street, Bristol BS1 2LY

common finding in the population. Longitudinal studies show that the prevalence of signs and symptoms of TMD increases with age and that the prevalence of signs is greater than the prevalence of symptoms. It has a variable incidence in an adolescent population between 5–35%.[5]

Most of the attempts at relating TMD to orthodontic treatment have been based on anecdotal evidence or retrospective studies, approaches that cannot demonstrate a cause and effect relationship between treatment and disease. An opinion held by a few was that occlusal interferences induced by orthodontic treatment would lead to TMD. This extended to the suggestion that orthodontic treatment is needed for those whose occlusion is not functionally optimal to prevent the development of TMD. A functional occlusion was defined as one in which intercuspal position should coincide with retruded contact position, there should not be any balancing side interferences and there should be anterior and canine guidance. Guidelines such as these are often referred to as treating to a 'functionally optimal occlusion' and were advocated by a group of 'functional orthodontists'. One viewpoint from a group of 'functional orthodontists' is that when premolar teeth are extracted for orthodontic treatment this leads to TMD because of over retracting the upper incisors during space closure, forcing the condyle into a posterior position. It is this posterior position of the condyle within the fossa, which is presumed to cause an anteriorly displaced disc and therefore TMD.[6] It was also believed that occlusal interferences would lead to TMD, as well as tooth wear, periodontal disease and instability of tooth position after orthodontic treatment if the position of the condyle was not 'rear most, mid most and upper most'. Roth demonstrated that the symptoms of TMD could be resolved once they were equilibrated with occlusal positioning splints.[7] However, these conclusions were reached after Roth had evaluated only nine patients post treatment and two of these acted as controls.

The debate concerning a relationship between orthodontic treatment and TMD came to a head in 1987 following a lawsuit, Brimm vs Malloy, in which it was claimed that orthodontic treatment had caused TMD in a patient. During the trial, the lack of good scientific evidence investigating the effects of orthodontic treatment and TMD was highlighted and prompted the formation of the American Association of Orthodontics Temporo Mandibular Joint Research Programme. This is perhaps the first time that orthodontists realised the lack of objective, scientific research into the effects of orthodontic treatment. Only recently has stronger evidence been forthcoming in assessing the role of orthodontic treatment with respect to TMD.

A number of studies have examined the position of the condyle and its relationship with TMD. They found that individuals with 'normal' joints (ie none have reported any signs or symptoms of TMD) had condyles that could be observed, randomly distributed, in anterior, centric and posterior positions in the glenoid fossa.[8] A posterior position of the condyle within the glenoid fossa cannot therefore be taken as proof of TMD.

When orthodontic treatment involves the extraction of upper first premolar teeth and the retraction of the upper incisors some have suggested that this predisposes the patient to TMD by posteriorly positioning the condyle. Some light has been shed on this position in a study of 42 patients with a Class II Division 1 malocclusion treated by the extraction of both upper first premolars and fixed appliances. Seventy per cent showed a forward movement of mandibular basal bone and the changes in condylar position did not correlate with incisor retraction (ie orthodontic treatment caused a transitory forward position of the condyle in the intercuspal position with a return to the pretreatment position after treatment). It was therefore concluded that orthodontic treatment involving the loss of premolar teeth did not cause TMD and this has been supported by the finding of other workers.[9,10]

The suggestion that orthodontic treatment causes a posteriorly positioned condyle, which in turn leads to TMD, appears to be ill founded. The clinical studies published so far conclude that orthodontic treatment has no role in worsening or causing TMD when treated patients are compared to untreated patients with or without a malocclusion.[11]

The final question that should be addressed is the need to treat our orthodontic cases to a 'functionally optimal occlusion'. There is little clinical evidence to suggest that such an occlusion has any benefits in terms of reducing the following:

- Tooth wear
- TMD
- Periodontal disease
- Instability of tooth position

Indeed intercuspal position rarely coincides with retruded contact position in a good occlusion and it has yet to be shown that canine guidance has an effect of preventing or curing TMD. A natural dentition with canine guidance will tend to become group functioning with time as the canines wear. Furthermore canine guidance does not seem to offer any protection against TMD.[12]

Although canine guidance is often advocated as the functioning mode of choice, it is often an unobtainable aim for a substantial proportion of orthodontic patients. A study investigating the frequency of group function and canine guidance patterns of occlusion as related to the Frankfort-mandibular plane angle found the following. It showed a positive relationship between canine guidance and low Frankfort-mandibular plane angles and of group function to high Frankfort-mandibular plane angles.[13] This would suggest that facial morphology may indicate which functional goal to aim for.

There are no clear occlusal objectives for orthodontic treatment although there are many occlusal goals which have been suggested. Occlusal goals are those directed at the relationship of the teeth both in static intercuspal position and during function. Andrews introduced his six keys to a normal occlusion as a means of obtaining a static intercuspal position that is seen as ideal.[14] A summary of these six keys is given below:

- Class I molar relationship
- Correct crown angulation
- Correct crown inclination
- No rotated teeth
- No interdental spaces
- Flat occlusal plane

In practice, orthodontically treated occlusions seldom achieve all occlusal keys because of differences in skeletal pattern and tooth size discrepancies.[15] It has however been shown that well intercuspated teeth may be more stable and less likely to relapse.[16]

There is a general agreement that intercuspal position should coincide with retruded contact position although there is a disagreement as to how closely they should coincide. The majority of the population have been shown to exhibit a discrepancy between the two positions with no ill effects. It seems sensible therefore to accept small discrepancies of approximately 1 mm or so of each other.

Summary of orthodontics and TMD
- Extracting teeth does not cause a posteriorly positioned condyle
- Orthodontics does not cause TMD

THE EXTRACTION VERSUS NON-EXTRACTION DEBATE

The extraction of teeth as part of orthodontic treatment continually causes controversy. Teeth are extracted for several reasons in orthodontics. The most common reason for extraction is the relief of crowding and the need to create space to gain good alignment of the teeth. The reduction of overbite and the correction of an increased overjet to obtain a Class I incisor relationship are also important issues to consider where extractions will be required.

Edward Angle was very influential during the 1890s in developing orthodontics as a speciality, with himself as the 'father of modern orthodontics'. He is credited with much of the development in the concept of occlusion in the natural dentition and a classification of malocclusion.

Angle believed in non-extraction orthodontic treatment and that every person had the potential for an ideal relationship of all 32 teeth. He was also concerned with the ideal facial aesthetics which he felt could be achieved when the dental arches had been expanded so that all the teeth were in ideal occlusion. Angle did not come to this expansion philosophy through clinical research but was convinced by the ideas of influential people of his time, namely Rousseau and Wolff. It was felt by Rousseau, a philosopher, that many of the ills of modern man were due to the environment we now live in and emphasised the 'perfectibility of man'. Therefore from an orthodontic perspective, a perfect occlusion could never be achieved by the extraction of teeth. In the early 1900s Wolff, a physiologist, demonstrated that remodelling of bone could occur in response to functional loading. Angle therefore reasoned that if teeth were placed in a proper occlusion, forces transmitted to the teeth would cause bone to grow around them. He went as far as describing his edgewise appliance as the 'bone growing appliance'. Any relapse seen in any of his treated cases was attributed to an inadequate occlusion.

It was not until the 1930s and the 1940s that this non-extraction rule advocated by Angle was challenged by Tweed and Begg. They both felt that a malocclusion was an inherited condition and dismissed the notion about the 'perfectibility of man'. Tweed argued about the poor long term stability of expanded dental arches and decided to retreat many of Angles cases by extracting four first premolars. He publicly demonstrated 100 consecutively treated patients claiming a more stable occlusion after extraction based treatment. An appliance system was created by Begg, which was designed to be used on extraction based treatments, which popularised this treatment approach.

The extraction debate has reopened recently, especially in North America, because of concerns of litigation if extraction based treatment philosophies are used. In recent years there has been a trend towards non-extraction treatment as studies have shown that even cases treated with the extraction of first premolars are not guaranteed a stable result.[17]

Summary of the extraction versus non-extraction debate
- Changing trends over the years in extraction/ non-extraction based treatment
- Arch expansion shows worst levels of relapse
- Extracting teeth does not guarantee future stability
- Each case should be properly treatment planned to give greatest future stability

DOES EXTRACTING TEETH DAMAGE FACES?

Some practitioners in recent years have shown anecdotal evidence that extracting teeth for orthodontic purposes ruins a patient's profile and compromises their facial aesthetics. It has been claimed that the orthodontic extraction of teeth may cause less attractive smiles with dark buccal spaces lateral to the buccal segments, known as the 'dark buccal corridor', and also by the retraction of the upper incisors when closing

Orthodontic treatment on an extraction or non-extraction basis will still show some relapse in most cases

the remaining extraction spaces giving a 'dished in' aged appearance.

These practitioners advocate a non-extraction approach to treatment on the basis that it will produce a more youthful, protrusive facial profile – a view held by Angle some one hundred years ago. The opinion that non-extraction treatment is better than extraction treatment when assessing facial attractiveness is clearly misinformed given the studies that have now been carried out.

There is a relationship between retraction of the upper incisors and the posterior movement of the upper lip but for any given individual this is unpredictable. Indeed, when the upper incisors are retracted by 5 mm it has been shown there is on average 1.4 mm posterior movement of the upper lip.[9] Those patients treated on an extraction basis have been found to have slightly more prominent lips compared with those treated on a non-extraction basis at the end of treatment.[18,19] It is of note to mention that in the extraction group they tended to have more prominent lips before commencing treatment because of an increased overjet, an important consideration when treatment planning these patients. There are many patients who have been treated on a non-extraction basis with a 'dished in' appearance and many other patients with fuller profiles who have had four teeth extracted as part of their orthodontic treatment. An important consideration before deciding on whether treatment is going to proceed on an extraction or non-extraction basis is the profile of the patient before treatment. It is important at this initial stage of assessment and planning to identify which patients are vulnerable to worsening an already flat or 'dished in' profile as they may not be amenable to orthodontic treatment alone and may require a combined surgical and orthodontic approach.

A question frequently raised is that of the differences in facial appearance if the same mildly crowded case was treated on an extraction or non-extraction basis. What would we expect to see at the end of treatment? One such retrospective study has addressed these issues by analysing the impact of extractions on the lip morphology in borderline Class II Division 1 malocclusions. In the extraction group where four first premolars were removed the lower incisors were on average 2 mm posterior and the lower lip 1.2 mm posterior when compared with a non-extraction group. It was seen that the non-extraction group had 2 mm fuller profile, although both groups were happy with their aesthetic appearance.[19]

Clinicians tend to be very critical about the changes, both in terms of the hard and soft tissues, which are brought about as a result of orthodontic treatment whether or not extractions have been carried out. Therefore the general public's perception about the profile of our patients after treatment should be given some thought. A timely and relevant study of the public's perception of the changes in profile of patients treated for a Class II Division 1 malocclusion concluded that they preferred the profile changes more in the extraction group compared with the non-extraction group. There was no preference for the profiles for either group two years after treatment.[20] It would seem then that there is no evidence to suggest that extraction based treatment when prescribed correctly 'damages faces'.

> **Summary of extracting teeth and damaged faces**
> - No evidence to suggest that extracting teeth in appropriate cases causes a 'dished in' appearance
> - Lay opinion finds both extraction and non-extraction treatment equally pleasing

SHOULD WE EXTRACT SECOND MOLARS AS PART OF ORTHODONTIC TREATMENT?

There are said to be many advantages in extracting second molars as part of orthodontic treatment. These advantages include the following:

- Less detrimental to facial profile
- Facilitates the eruption of third molars
- Spontaneous relief of crowding in the premolar region
- Prevents crowding in a well aligned lower arch
- Aids distal movement of the buccal segments with extra oral traction
- Shorter treatment time
- Functional occlusion is better

It can be seen that it is an impressive list of advantages! There are however several considerations that need to be taken into account before extracting second molar teeth with radiological evaluation of third molar development essential. All third molars should be present, and have good size, shape and position.

The idea that extracting second molars is less detrimental to the facial profile is an interesting concept, given that the tooth to be extracted is in a more posterior position in the mouth compared to premolar teeth and is therefore thought less likely to adversely affect soft tissue profile. One study investigated this claim by comparing the effects different extraction patterns on the facial profile between two groups, those treated by first premolar extraction and another by second molar extraction. They found the average decrease in the soft tissue angle of facial convexity of 1.7° for the second molar extraction group and 2.2° for the first premolar group. However, these reductions were not statistically significant and it must be remembered that these patients were not derived from the same population, as they were not randomised to one of the extraction patterns.[21]

The ideal time for extracting second molars is controversial, some studies have suggested the best time to extract them is when the third

Lay populations and patients cannot perceive significant profile changes after appropriate orthodontic treatment which may or may not involve orthodontic extractions

molar crown is fully formed and others claim they should be extracted as soon as they erupt into the mouth. The evidence suggests that the importance of timing second molar extractions is not yet known. One disadvantage of extracting second molars is the 'predictably unpredictable' nature of third molar development and eruption. A number of studies have shown that third molar eruption is often unsatisfactory including improper angulation and contact relationship with the first molar. This is seen ranging from 4–25% of cases[22] and raises doubts on the length of treatment time for second molar extraction cases compared to other extraction strategies. The loss of second molar teeth obviates the need for space closing mechanics but a second course of treatment may be required to orthodontically upright third molars at a stage in late adolescence when co-operation may not be at its best.

An important reason for elective extractions in orthodontics is the relief of crowding. First premolar teeth are ideally located as they provide up to 14 mm of space for the relief of crowding both anteriorly and posteriorly to the extraction site. Second molar teeth can provide some 18–22 mm of space, of which little is made available to the relief of crowding in the lower labial segment where crowding most often occurs. Given that arch length deficiencies rarely exceed 10 mm the removal of a second molar tooth and the space it provides seems a little excessive. However, if the premolar region is crowded by 4–5 mm then the removal of second molar teeth may provide sufficient space for spontaneous relief of premolar crowding. The relief of molar crowding in the early permanent dentition is an indication to extract second molars and it may also prevent late lower arch crowding.[23]

Many of the advantageous claims made for the extraction of second molar teeth are unsubstantiated. There is no evidence to suggest that treatment times are shorter, that distal movement of the first maxillary molar is enhanced and that there is less effect on the soft tissue profile. The benefits of extracting second molars appear to be relief of mild premolar crowding in the early permanent dentition but eruption of the third molar needs careful review and the possibility of a later additional course of orthodontic treatment needs to be made clear to the patients.

Summary on the extraction of second molars

- Many of the claimed advantages are unsubstantiated
- Evidence suggests relief of molar and premolar crowding is an indication
- Third molar development is 'predictably unpredictable' and may need further treatment to orthodontically upright them

---

THE 'ORTHOPAEDIC EFFECT' — CAN WE INFLUENCE GROWTH?

The potential to influence growth, whether it is promoting growth in a Class II malocclusion or restricting growth in a Class III malocclusion, remains an area of significant controversy. A number of studies have looked into the possibility of modifying growth with orthopaedic appliances and the results are liberally interpreted to suit the position of the challenger. An 'orthopaedic effect' is taken to mean a change in the position of the cranio-facial skeleton in relation to each other as the result of orthodontic treatment. This change should be permanent in its amount and direction.

Functional appliances have been used for many years for the correction of Class II malocclusions. Despite this long history there continues to be much debate relating to their use, mode of action and effectiveness. Undoubtedly, normal dentofacial growth has a genetic drive but maybe influenced by environmental factors. There is no doubt that functional appliances can rapidly correct Class II malocclusion but this does not indicate or prove an 'orthopaedic effect'.

Some practitioners like to claim they can 'grow mandibles', but what is their evidence? Many studies find an increase in mandibular length of 1–2 mm per annum during active treatment.[24] Much of the work demonstrating the ability of functional appliances to stimulate mandibular growth is based on animal experimentation. A maximum of 5–15% increase in mandibular length by stimulating condylar growth can be expected in experimental animals under controlled conditions and during periods of active growth.[25] Animal experimental research is often cited as evidence but cautious interpretation of the results is required before it is applied to patients.

There is evidence from prospective randomised controlled trials that the effects of functional appliances maybe transient, with reversion to pretreatment growth patterns over the short or long term.[26] Therefore this short-term growth enhancement is useful to correct incisor and molar relationships but does not result in a longer mandible. They produce their effects mainly by dentoalveolar changes such as retroclination of upper incisors and proclination of the lower incisors.[27]

An orthopaedic change has also been attempted in Class III malocclusions where it is largely assumed that the fault lies with a prognathic mandible. Hence chin cup treatment, once popular, was directed at restraining further mandibular growth and allowing maxillary growth to 'catch up' and therefore correct the anterioposterior component of a Class III malocclusion. A long-term study looking at the effect of chin cup therapy found that it was effective in reducing mandibular prognathism before puberty but this was then lost after puberty ie a short-term gain similar to that seen with functional appliances. Indeed, there was no difference in

> The orthodontist's ability to influence facial growth is limited and much of the change that is seen relates to dento alveolar changes

the final skeletal profile of the mandible between treatment groups and control groups who did not receive treatment.[28]

However, there appears to be a promising method of achieving an 'orthopaedic effect' with the use of protraction headgear. Several workers have shown that a small but significant anterior movement of the maxillae using protraction headgear during the mixed dentition is possible which has remained stable some 2 years after treatment.[29]

In summary, orthodontic appliances that deliver an orthopaedic effect may induce a temporary improvement in the skeletal relationship. There is no evidence at present to show that orthodontic treatment can effectively restrain or enhance cranio-facial growth that is otherwise inherited by the individual.[30]

Summary of the current evidence on the 'orthopaedic effect'
- Orthodontic treatment cannot influence growth in the long term
- Any gain is small but is often lost in the long term
- Majority of the 'orthopaedic effect' is dentoalveolar tipping of the teeth

---

We have chosen four areas of smouldering controversy not to rekindle historic arguments or generate a new turf war but to illustrate the somewhat flimsy evidence both sides of an argument can use. Forceful opinion currently dominates any cautious interpretation of the existing literature. Given time, the quality of the data and research will improve and as a consequence more definitive statements on true effects of treatment will be possible.

1. Haynes R B, Richardson W S. Evidence based medicine: what it is and what it isn't. *Br Med J* 1996; **312:** 71-72.
2. Richards D, Lawrence A. Evidence based dentistry. *Br Dent J* 1995; **179:** 270-273.
3. Harrison J E. Ashby D. Orthodontic treatment for posterior crossbites (Cochrane Review). *Cochrane Database Syst Rev* 2001; **1:** CD000979.
4. Burke S P, Silveira A M, Goldsmith L J, Yancey J M, Van Stewart A, Scarfe W C. A meta-analysis of mandibular intercanine width in treatment and postretention. *Angle Orthod* 1998; **68:** 53-60.
5. Proffit W. *Contemporary Orthodontics.* 3rd ed. St Lewis: Mosby-Year book, 1999.
6. Witzig J W, Spahl T J. *The clinical management of basic maxillofacial orthopaedic appliances.* Vol 2 Diagnosis. pp221-224. Boston: PSG Publishing, 1987.
7. Roth R. Temporomandibular pain-dysfunction and occlusal relationships. *Angle Orthod* 1973; **43:** 136-153.
8. Ren Y F. *et al.* Condyle position in the temporomandibular joint. Comparison between asymptomatic volunteers with normal disk position and patients with disk displacement. *Oral Surg, Oral Med, Oral Path, Oral Radiol, Endo* 1995; **80:** 101-107.
9. Lueke P E, Johnston L E. The effect of first premolar extraction and incisor retraction on mandibular positions: testing the central dogma of 'functional orthodontics'. *Am J Orthod Dentofac Orthop* 1992; **101:** 4-12.
10. Gianelly A A. *et al.* Condylar position and maxillary first premolar extraction. *Am J Orthod Dentofac Orthop* 1991; **99:** 473-476.
11. Luther F. Orthodontics and the temporomandibular joint: Where are we now? *Angle Orthod* 1998; **68:** 295-317.
12. Bush F M. Malocclusion, masticatory muscle and temporomandibular joint tenderness. *J Dent Res* 1985; **64:** 129-133.
13. DiPetro G J. A study of occlusion as related to the Frankfort-mandibular plane angle. *J Prosthetic Dent* 1977; **38:** 452-458.
14. Andrews L F. The six keys to normal occlusion. *Am J Orthod* 1972; **62:** 296-309.
15. Kattner P F, Schneider B J. Comparision of Roth appliance and standard edgewise appliance treatment results. *Am J Orthod Dentofac Orthop* 1993; **103:** 24-32.
16. Lloyd T G, Stephens C D. Changes in molar occlusion after extraction of all first premolars: A follow up study of Class II division 1 cases treated wth removable appliances. *Br J Ortho* 1990; **6:** 91-94.
17. Little R M. An evaluation of changes in mandibular anterior alignment from 10 to 20 years postretention. *Am J Orthod* 1988; **93:** 423-428.
18. James R D. A comparative study of facial profiles in extraction and nonextraction treatment. *Am J Orthod Dentofac Orthop* 1998; **114:** 265-276.
19. Paquette D E *et al.* A long term comparison of nonextraction and premolar extraction edgewise therapy in 'boderline' Class II patients. *Am J Orthod Dentofac Orthop* 1992; **102:** 1-14
20. Bishara S E., Jakobsen J R. Profile changes in patients treated with and without extractions: Assessments by lay people. *Am J Orthod Dentofac Orthop* 1997; **112:** 639-644.
21. Staggers J A. A comparison of second molar and first premolar extraction treatment. *Am J Orthod Dentofac Orthop* 1990; **98:** 430-436.
22. Gooris C G M. *et al.* Eruption of third molars after second molar extractions: A radiographic study. *Am J Orthod Dentofac Orthop* 1990; **98:** 161-167.
23. Richardson M E. Lower molar crowding in the early permanent dentition. *Angle Orthod* 1985; **55:** 51-57.
24. Lagerstrom L. Dental and skeletal contributions to occlusal correction in patients treated with high pull headgear-activator combination. *Am J Orthod Dentofac Orthop* 1990; **97:** 495-504.
25. McNamara J A. Skeletal and dental changes following functional regulator therapy on class II patients. *Am J Orthod* 1985; **88:** 91-110.
26. De Vincenzo J P. Changes in mandibular length before during and after successful orthopaedic correction of Class II malocclusion using a functional appliance. *Am J Orthod Dentofac Orthop* 1991; **99:** 214-257.
27. Bishara S E. Functional Appliances: A review. *Am J Orthod Dentofac Orthop* 1989; **95:** 250-258.
28. Suagawara J. Long term effects of chincap therapy on skeletal profile in mandibular prognathism. *Am J Orthod Dentofac Orthop* 1990; **98:** 127-133.
29. Ngan P. Cephalometric and occlusal changes following maxillary protraction and expansion. *Eur J Orthod* 1998; **20:** 237-254.
30. Chate R A. The burden of proof: a critical review of orthodontic claims made by some general practitioners. *Am J Orthod Dentofac Orthop* 1994; **106:** 96-105.

IN BRIEF

- The extraction of teeth for orthodontic purposes has always been a controversial area. It is not possible to treat all malocclusions without taking out teeth
- Where extractions are indicated, first premolars are most commonly extracted but there are reasons for extracting elsewhere in the arch and this will involve other teeth
- The use of fixed appliances has considerably changed extraction viewpoints

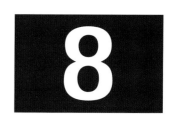

Extractions in orthodontics

H. Travess*, D. Roberts-Harry and J. Sandy

Extractions in orthodontics remains a relatively controversial area. It is not possible to treat all malocclusions without taking out any teeth. The factors which affect the decision to extract include the patient's medical history, the attitude to treatment, oral hygiene, caries rates and the quality of teeth. Extractions of specific teeth are required in the various presentations of malocclusion. In some situations careful timing of extractions may result in spontaneous correction of the malocclusion.

*Senior Specialist Registrar in Orthodontics, Division of Child Dental Health, University of Bristol Dental School, Lower Maudlin Street, Bristol BS1 2LY

The role of extractions in orthodontic treatment has been a controversial subject for over a century. It is fair to say that even today, opinion is divided on whether extractions are used too frequently in the correction of malocclusion.

Angle[1] believed that all 32 teeth could be accommodated in the jaws, in an ideal occlusion with the first molars in a Class I occlusion, ie with the mesiobuccal cusp of the upper first molar occluding in the buccal groove of the lower first molar. Extraction was anathema to his ideals, as he believed bone would form around the teeth in their new position, according to Wolff's law.[2] This was criticised in 1911 by Case who believed extractions were necessary in order to relieve crowding and aid stability of treatment.[3]

Two of Angle's students at around the same time but in different countries considered the need for extractions in achieving stable results. Tweed became disappointed in the results he was achieving and decided to re-treat a number of patients who had suffered relapse following orthodontic treatment (at no further cost) using extraction of four premolar units.[4]

The demonstration of his results to the profession in America resulted in a change of philosophy in the 1940s to extraction-based techniques. Begg, in Australia, studied Aboriginal skulls and noted a large amount of occlusal and more importantly interproximal wear.[5] He argued that premolar extractions were required in order to compensate for the lack of interproximal wear seen in the modern Australian dentition, through lack of a coarse diet. He also developed a technique that relied on extractions to create much of the anchorage needed for treatment.

Recently, the extraction debate has reopened, with some individuals believing that expansion of the jaws and retraining of posture can obviate the need for extractions and produce stable results. These claims are for the most part unsubstantiated. If teeth are genuinely crowded as opposed to being irregular then arch alignment can be achieved by one of the following:

- Enlargement of the archform
- Reduction in tooth size
- Reduction in tooth number

Arch expansion can be achieved by moving teeth buccally and labially (ie lateral and anterio posterior expansion) but the long-term stability and whether bone grows as teeth are moved through cortical plates remain contentious issues. In the maxilla there is a suture which remains patent in some patients into the second decade. This can also be used in expansion in that it can be 'split' with rapid maxillary expansion. The split suture fills in with bone and thus a wider arc to accommodate teeth is created. There is no good evidence that this method of expansion produces a more stable result than any other method. Longitudinal studies provide useful guidance on whether arch expansion produces stability. These are difficult studies to conduct but increasing mandibular length to accommodate teeth relapses in nearly 90% of cases with resulting unsatisfactory anterior tooth alignment.[6]

Reduction in tooth size particularly in the labial segments with interdental stripping is another potential mechanism to relieve crowding. Variable relapse has been reported but one study noted relapse of some degree in all cases.[7]

This work was done over 25 years ago and does not reflect contemporary use of inter-dental enamel reduction or current retention regimes.

The reduction in tooth number is usually achieved with extractions and these cases ideally need to be compared with treated non extraction cases with spacing, cases treated by arch expansion to accommodate crowding and untreated normal occlusions. In a review of these issues it was concluded that arch length reduces in most cases, including untreated normal occlusion. Any lateral expansion across the mandibular canines decreases after treatment but this is also seen in those cases which have no orthodontic treatment. It was further recognised that mandibular anterior crowding is a continuing phenomenon seen in patients into the fourth decade and likely beyond.[8] The degree of anterior crowding seen at the end of retention is variable and unpredictable.

Proffit[9] in a 40-year review of extraction patterns showed 30% of cases were treated with extractions in 1953, 76% in 1968 and 28% in 1993. He suggested the decline in extractions since 1968 was because of concern over facial profile, tempromandibular joint dysfunction (TMD) and stability; the change from the Begg appliance, largely an extraction-based technique to the straight wire technique, which seems to require fewer extractions. The latter may also result with a change in mindset and the use of headgear and prolonged retention.

A dogmatic approach is inadvisable and each case must be assessed on its merits. Some cases, especially where the crowding is mild may not need tooth removal, and a more sensible approach based on the requirements of the individual case rather that the two extremes seen in the past century is advised. Interestingly, in a follow up study over a 15 year period in Scotland, orthodontics replaced caries as the commonest reason for extraction in patients under 20 years of age.[10] All extractions are traumatic as far as the patient is concerned and clinicians will seek non-extraction solutions where possible. In the late mixed dentition, between 3 mm and 4 mm of space can be preserved in the lower arch by simply fitting a lingual arch. If this is coupled with molar and premolar expansion of just 2 mm (with no lower canine exapansion) and interdental enamel reduction between anterior contact points then a large proportion of otherwise 'crowded' cases can be treated without the loss of permanent teeth. The decision on whether or not to extract teeth is based on an assessment of many factors including crowding, increase in overjet, change in arch width, curve of Spee, anchorage requirements and other more esoteric factor such as adjusting the torque of the anterior teeth. It is also worth mentioning that the concept of space analysis is probably under used in the United Kingdom, but this is routinely applied elsewhere. This analysis enables a rationale and methodical approach to treatment planning before extractions are recommended.[11] It is important then to realise that there are a variety of options as far as mild to moderate crowding cases are concerned.

FACTORS AFFECTING THE DECISION TO EXTRACT

It is important to consider the patient as a whole in treatment planning. Medical history, attitude to treatment, oral hygiene, caries rate and the quality of the teeth are important. Patients with cardiac anomalies are at risk of complications during orthodontic treatment and consultation with a cardiologist is important. If necessary, extractions should be covered with appropriate antibiotics and impacted teeth may be best removed rather than aligned as traction to unerupted teeth may pose an increased risk to these patients.[12]

The quality and prognosis of the teeth should be carefully considered, as this may override other factors. Hypoplastic, heavily restored or carious teeth should generally be removed in preference to healthy teeth. This is especially true in the labial segments where aesthetics are difficult to maintain with loss of an incisor or canine.

Teeth of abnormal form or size may be considered for removal as they can look unsightly and be difficult to align. For example, a dens-indente may compromise the long-term prognosis of a tooth, or a talon cusp may hinder arch co-ordination during treatment. Dilacerated teeth should be carefully assessed to see if crown alignment is achievable. Often extraction of these teeth is the only option. Macrodont teeth, geminated or fused, need careful consideration (Fig. 1). The aesthetics are often poor but extraction can result in an excess amount of space, which may prolong orthodontic treatment. Where supplemental teeth are present, extraction may result in spontaneous correction of any crowding (Fig. 2).

Fig. 1 Illustration of a macrodont tooth in the lower labial segment, which also exhibits a talon cusp. Alignment and arch co-ordination is hindered by the size of the tooth and the talon cusp. Some enamel reduction can be undertaken to reduce the width of the tooth but care must be taken not to breach the enamel. In the upper arch, reduction of a talon cusp can help correct an increased overjet, although radiographic examination of pulp chambers in the talon cusp is essential

EASE OF EXTRACTION, AND THE PRESENCE OF IMPACTED TEETH

The extraction of teeth is a potentially traumatic experience. The decision to extract should be made with an awareness of the risks of treatment, including the psychological impact of the procedure. The General Dental Council in its guidance to dentists of professional and personal conduct makes it clear that dentists who refer patients for general anaesthesia must make it clear what justification there is for the procedure. The duties of the treating dentist include a thorough and clear explanation of the risks involved as well as the alternative methods of pain control available. The use of general anaesthesia is usually considered in dealing with unerupted teeth, first molars, multiple extractions in four quadrants and specific phobias.

If teeth are impacted or ectopically positioned, extraction of an erupted tooth can guide the path of eruption of the impacted tooth and obviate the need for minor oral surgery. For example, the impaction of a lower second premolar may be relieved by the removal of the first premolar or first molar, which only requires local analgesia and is less traumatic than the removal of the impacted tooth (Fig. 3). In Figure 4, eruption of the upper second premolars resulted in severe resorption of the roots of the upper first molars. Extracting these molars would be fairly atraumatic and allow the second premolars to erupt into the mouth. Similarly, if unerupted permanent canines are palatally positioned judicious removal of the deciduous canines can improve the path of eruption of the permanent teeth and may help to avoid lengthy orthodontic treatment.[13]

CORRECTION OF OVERBITE

Space closure with fixed appliances tends to increase the overbite and therefore extractions in the lower arch in deep bite cases should be undertaken with caution. In some malocclusions, where the anterior face height is reduced, extractions can make space closure difficult and great care must be taken in diagnosis before this decision is made. It is important to recognise whether a case is genuinely crowded or whether the teeth are displaced lingually as in a Class II Division 2 case. Lingually displaced lower labial segments are frequently not crowded, even though they may appear to be so.

Proclination of the lower labial segment also reduces the overbite, as well as overjet, and may obviate the need for extractions. However, this treatment approach should be undertaken cautiously as uncontrolled and excessive proclination of the lower incisors can be unstable and should only be undertaken in selected cases by experienced clinicians. Flattening of an accentuated curve of Spee in order to reduce an overbite, where proclination is contraindicated, does require space, for which the extraction of lower teeth can sometimes be considered. The space required to flatten a curve of Spee has historically been over rated, the amount of space required is

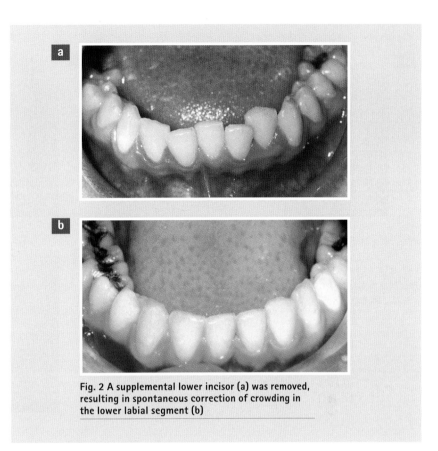

Fig. 2 A supplemental lower incisor (a) was removed, resulting in spontaneous correction of crowding in the lower labial segment (b)

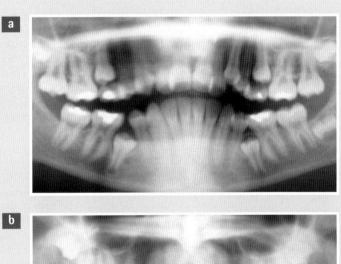

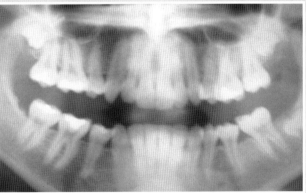

Fig. 3 This case presented with missing upper first premolars and lower right third molar, with vertically impacted lower second premolars. (a) Both lower first molars are heavily filled and would be ideal for extraction to allow eruption of the second premolars. However the missing third molar on the right resulted in extraction of the lower right first premolar and the lower left first molar. Spontaneous alignment occurred (b) with both impacted premolars erupting successfully into the occlusion with no active treatment

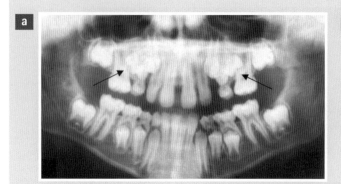
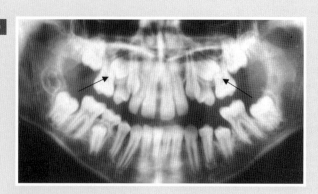

Fig. 4 In this case, the erupting upper second premolars showed some resorption of the mesial roots of the upper first molars. (a) Progressive resorption of the mesial roots of the molars was seen on subsequent radiographs (b), which progressed to such an extent (c) that both upper first molars required extraction, allowing eruption of the second premolars

1–2 mm when the curve is severe and there is no crowding. It is difficult then to justify extracting teeth purely for the sake of creating space to flatten an occlusal curve. The greatest challenge is the mechanical control of the teeth to prevent excessive proclination of the lower incisors. This usually occurs because the intrusion force is at some distance labial to the centre of resistance of the incisors and lingual crown torque is needed to prevent the labial movement of the incisors.

EXTRACTION OF SPECIFIC TEETH

Despite the factors discussed above, certain teeth are extracted preferentially for orthodontic reasons. A survey of extraction patterns in the hospital orthodontic service (Table 1) showed that first premolars were most commonly extracted (59%) followed by second premolars (13%). Permanent molars accounted for 19% of extractions (12% for first molars and 7% for second molars). Only 1% of patients had incisor extractions.[14]

The high percentage of premolar extractions is related to their position in the arch and the

timing of their eruption. They are often ideal for the relief of anterior and posterior crowding. However, each patient should be seen as an individual and their treatment planned according to the merits of the malocclusion,

Lower incisors

In general, removal of a lower incisor should be avoided, as the inter-canine width tends to decrease which can result in crowding developing in the upper labial segment or the overjet increasing. However, a number of situations do exist in which a lower incisor may be considered as part of an orthodontic treatment plan and fixed appliances are generally required in these cases. These include situations where a lower incisor is grossly displaced from the arch form or 'ectopic' and space is required to align the teeth. This is best considered in adults and especially those who have had previous loss of premolar units in each quadrant and present with late lower labial segment crowding (Fig. 5). Class III cases at the limit of their growth can be camouflaged with loss of a lower incisor, to allow the lower labial segment to be tipped lingually, correcting the incisor relationship. This also tends to increase the overbite, which is helpful in these cases.[15] Treatment of Class I cases with moderate lower labial segment crowding of up to 5 mm (ie the size of a lower incisor) may be treated with loss of a lower incisor. An increase in overjet or a slightly Class III buccal segment relation may be an undesirable side effect.[16] Cases where a tooth size discrepancy exists, for example with upper peg shaped laterals or missing upper lateral incisors may also benefit from the loss of a lower incisor.

Table 1 Table of percentage extractions according to tooth type

Tooth	% removed
Central incisor	1
Lateral incisor	3
Canine	4
First premolar	59
Second premolar	13
First molar	12
Second molar	7

A Bolton analysis (a measure of tooth size discrepancies) may be used to analyse the extent of the disproportion. A Kesling set up[17] (where the anterior teeth are sectioned from a plaster model and re-positioned in wax as a trial set up, having left out a lower incisor) may be helpful in predicting the final outcome (Fig. 6).

Upper Incisors

Upper incisors are rarely the extraction of choice to treat a malocclusion. However, the upper labial segment is particularly at risk from trauma, especially in Class II Division 1 cases with large overjets. In situations where the long-term prognosis of an incisor is poor, for example, the incisor is non vital, root filled, dilacerated or of abnormal form, the tooth should be considered for extraction as part of the orthodontic treatment plan. Full consideration should be given to the resulting occlusion and aesthetics. Placing a lateral incisor in a central incisor position rarely gives a good result because the root of the tooth is narrow and the emergence angle of the built up crown is poor. In some cases transplantation of a premolar with a developing root into the incisor socket can relieve crowding in the lower arch and provide a useful replacement in the upper labial segment (Fig. 7).

Where lateral incisors are diminutive or missing, space closure or space maintenance can be considered more equally. Attention must be paid to the shape, size, gingival height and colour of the canine if a good aesthetic result is to be achieved. In many cases the canines can be disguised as lateral incisors by selective grinding, and where appropriate, aesthetic build-ups.

Canines

These teeth are rarely considered for extraction unless very ectopic (Fig. 8). The loss of a canine makes canine guidance impossible and may compromise a good functional occlusal result. Contact between a premolar and lateral incisor is often poor and canines can act as ideal abutment teeth because of their long root length and resistance to periodontal problems. Palatally ectopic canines can sometimes be in unfavourable positions for alignment, and lower ectopic canines often require extraction rather than alignment. In many of the former cases the first premolar can be aligned with a mesial inclination and rotated mesio-palatally to hide the palatal cusp and provide a better aesthetic result.

Premolars

Premolars are often ideal for the relief of both anterior and posterior crowding, the first and second premolars have similar crown forms, which means that an acceptable contact point can be achieved between the remaining premolar and the adjacent molar and canine. The choice between first or second premolar depends on a number of factors for example, the degree of crowding, the anchorage requirements, the overjet and overbite.

In Class I cases where crowding exists and the

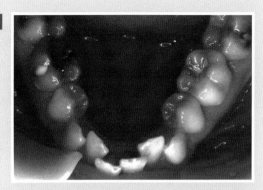

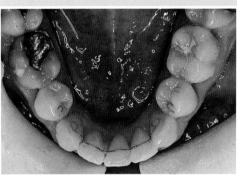

Fig. 5 Premolars had previously been extracted as part of orthodontic treatment in adolescence. Crowding returned in the lower labial segment (a), which was relieved by removal of a lower incisor and fixed appliance treatment. A bonded retainer was fitted at the completion of treatment (b)

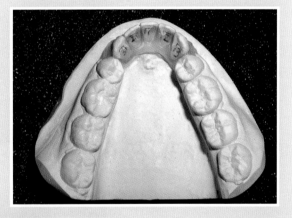

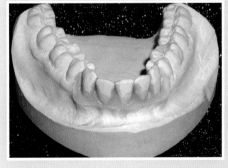

Fig. 6 A Kesling set up of the case in Figure 5, removing the lower left central incisor and replacing the remaining incisors and canines.
This showed the anticipated tooth positions and occlusion with the upper arch

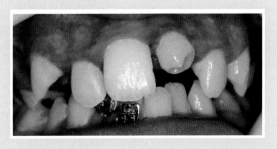

Fig. 7 A lower premolar has been transplanted to replace the upper left central incisor which had a poor prognosis

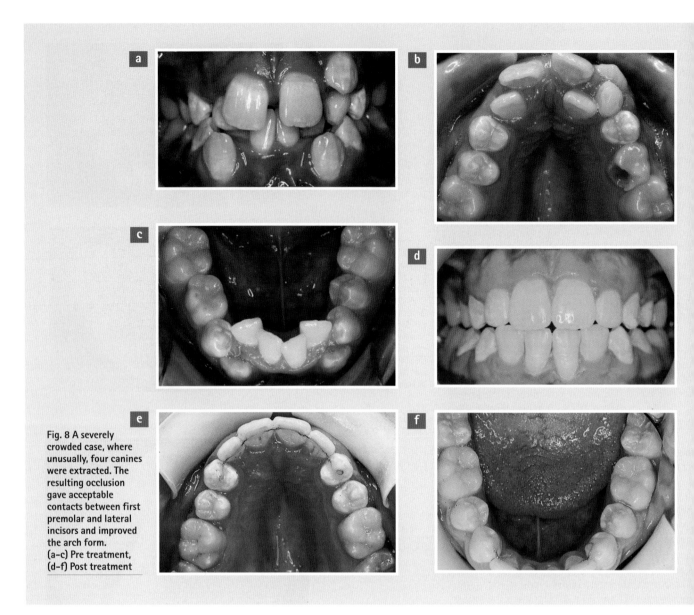

Fig. 8 A severely crowded case, where unusually, four canines were extracted. The resulting occlusion gave acceptable contacts between first premolar and lateral incisors and improved the arch form.
(a–c) Pre treatment,
(d–f) Post treatment

canines are mesially angulated, loss of first premolars may produce spontaneous improvement in the alignment of the canines (Fig. 9). Any excess extraction spaces may close with time, although a study by Berg *et al.*, showed space closure to be greatest in the first 6 months following extraction.[18] In carefully selected cases reasonable alignment can sometimes be achieved. However cases amenable to this type of treatment are rare and fixed appliances especially when second premolars have been extracted invariably produce better results.

Second premolars are the third most commonly developmentally absent teeth after third molars and upper lateral incisors.[19] Where deciduous molars are retained beyond their normal exfoliation dates, a radiograph should be taken to confirm the presence and position of the permanent successor. In uncrowded arches deciduous molars with good roots are often retained, as space closure in these cases can be difficult (Fig. 10).

Second premolars can become impacted either due to early loss of deciduous molars or severe crowding. Ectopic second premolars usu-ally erupt lingually or palatally and should be considered for extraction if they are completely excluded from the arch (Fig. 11).

First molars

First permanent molars are often the first permanent teeth to erupt into the mouth. Their deep fissure morphology predisposes them to caries and poor tooth brushing combined with a high sugar intake, may result in gross caries. Heavily restored or decayed first molars should be considered for removal over other non-carious teeth (Fig. 12). First molars extraction requires careful planning. Their position in the arch means that whilst relief of premolar crowding is achieved the space created is far from the site of any incisor crowding or overjet reduction. The timing of the loss of first molars is also an important consideration.

Maxillary second molars have a curvilinear eruptive path with mesial and vertical components. The lower second molar has a more vertical path, but it has to move more horizontally in favourable spontaneous molar correction. This is one of the reasons why the spontaneous tooth

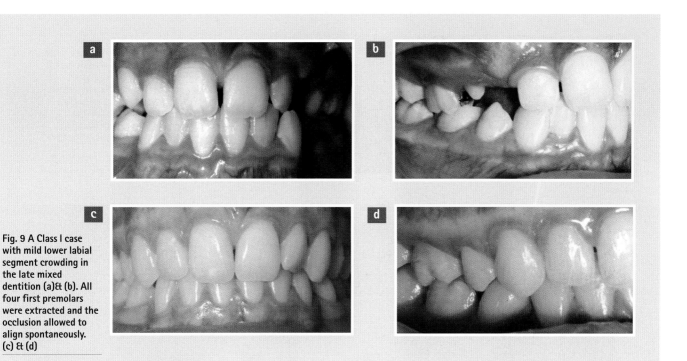

Fig. 9 A Class I case with mild lower labial segment crowding in the late mixed dentition (a) & (b). All four first premolars were extracted and the occlusion allowed to align spontaneously. (c) & (d)

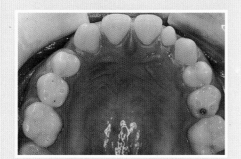

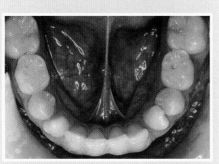

Fig. 10 A hypodontia case pre-treatment showing good quality deciduous molars which were retained as part of the treatment plan. Mesio-distal reduction or 'slenderising' can be used to maximise arch co-ordination, especially where deciduous molars are only retained in one arch

second premolar. Spontaneous relief of mild crowding in the labial segments may be seen. In the lower arch, spontaneous closure is less likely, but mesial migration of the second molar is also optimal at this stage and may resulting in minimal space between the second molar and second premolar (Fig. 12).

In the permanent dentition the effect of loss of a first molar can be difficult to predict after the second molar has erupted. Fixed appliances are invariably needed at this stage to align the teeth and achieve space closure with parallel roots.[20] The effects are more of a problem in the lower arch, where the second molar tips mesially and rolls lingually forming a very poor contact with the second premolar or may leave excess space. Little spontaneous relief of anterior crowding is seen. The upper first molar if retained can over-erupt, further increasing the tipping and rolling of the lower second molar. In addition mesial movement of the lower

movement is less favourable in the lower arch. Three periods of development can be considered when looking at the effects of loss of first molars.

Maximal space closure by mesial migration of the second molar occurs in the mixed dentition. At this stage the second molars are unerupted and their root furcation is just calcifying. The best results occur in the upper arch where the second molar usually will usually erupt mesially and make contact with the upper

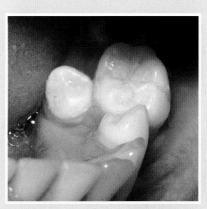

Fig. 11 Localised crowding often manifests in the lower buccal segments by lingual eruption of the second premolar

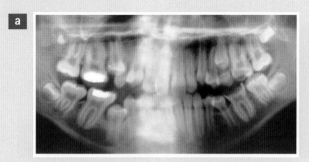

Fig. 12 Four first molars were extracted just after the optimal time, prior to fixed appliance treatment. The Orthopantomogram (a) shows gross caries in the left first molars and heavy restorations in the right first molars. Notice the discrepancy in space available in the two arches. In the upper arch the second molars have erupted in close proximity to the second premolars due to their mesial eruptive path (b). In the lower arch there is considerably more space remaining from the vertical eruptive path of the second molars (c)

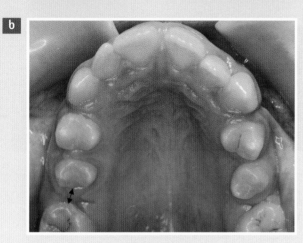

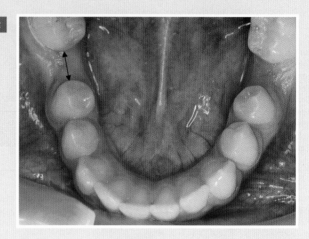

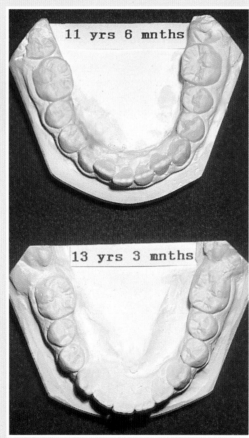

Fig. 13 Extraction of second molars allowed spontaneous relief of anterior crowding, with early eruption of the third molars

molar may be prevented. The upper second molar shows less tipping and rolling than its lower counterpart, but does not align to the extent seen in the mixed dentition. In adult patients the drifting of both upper and lower second molars is less marked, and the relief of crowding less reliable. In young patients, radiographs should be checked to ensure that the developing lower second premolar is contained by the roots of the primary molar. If not, then substantial drifting of the second premolar can take place including impaction into the mesial surface of the second molar.

In general terms if a lower first molar is to be extracted, the upper molar on the same side should also be extracted (compensating extraction). This prevents unwanted over-eruption of the upper first molar and the upper second molar will usually erupt into a good position. However, if an upper first molar is to be extracted, the lower counter-part is usually left *in situ*. This is because the lower second molar behaves unpredictably and rarely achieves good spontaneous alignment. An additional factor is that lower molars over erupt less than upper molars and will not interfere with the generally good progress made by upper second molars. If the case has no crowding, then balancing extractions should not be considered (removal of a tooth on the opposite side of the same arch). Children presenting with carious first molars often show signs of disease in all of them. If the timing is correct and the malocclusion justifies treatment, all four first molars should be removed to allow second molars to erupt efficiently and reduce subsequent treatment times.

Second molars

Thomas et al.[21] provided a succinct summary on the role of loss of second molars in orthodontic treatment. They state that all other teeth should be present with the third molars of normal size, shape and in a good position to erupt. Mild lower labial segment crowding may be effectively treated by loss of second molars, however they should not be considered in the treatment of moderate or severe crowding. Second molar loss may be undertaken under the following circumstances:

- To facilitate the eruption of the third molars obviating the need for surgical removal at a later stage.
- To allow relief of premolar crowding (especially where second premolars are impacted)
- May prevent crowding in a well-aligned lower arch (Fig. 13).
- Distal movement in the upper arch is more reliable and more stable.

However, the potential disadvantages of second molar extraction are:

- Eruption of third molars especially in the lower arch is unpredictable. About 30% of these teeth require uprighting.
- The teeth are remote from the site of crowding making alignment unpredictable.

Where second molars are considered for extraction, the timing is important. Satisfactory third molar alignment is less likely if the second molars are extracted after the third molar roots are more than one third formed.

Third molars

Whilst extraction of wisdom teeth for orthodontic purposes is rare, these teeth should be included in the treatment planning. The incidence of impaction of third molars varies widely in the literature.[22] Posterior crowding especially in the lower arch may increase the risk of developing impaction. Extraction of teeth towards the front of the mouth has little effect on posterior crowding, whilst extractions towards the back improve the chances of acceptable third molars eruption. The greatest benefit occurs when second molars are removed, although eruption patterns are unpredictable. Richardson et al.[23] suggest that up to 90% of third molars erupt into satisfactory positions following second molar removal, but this depends on the degree of posterior crowding and stage of root development of third molars at time of extraction. It also assumes a fairly broad minded view of what is a 'satisfactory' position.

Third molars have in the past been implicated in the aetiology of late lower incisor crowding.[23] However, more recent research shows that their presence is only one of the factors involved and their influence appears to be negligible. Therefore, third molars should not be removed to relieve or prevent late lower incisor crowding.[24] This forms part of the National Clinical Guidelines on the management of patients with impacted third molars.[22]

CONCLUSIONS

Many factors influence the choice of teeth for extraction and careful treatment planning in conjunction with good patient co-operation, appliance selection and management of the treatment are essential if an acceptable, aesthetic and functional occlusion is to be achieved.

1. Angle E H. Treatment of malocclusion of the teeth and fractures of the maxillae, Angle's system. Ed 6, 1900 S.S. Philadelphia: White Dental Manufacturing Co.
2. Wolff J. Das Gesetz der Transformation der Knochen. Berlin: Hirschwald, 1892.
3. Case C S. The question of extraction in orthdontia. Am J Orthod 1964; **50:** 658-691.
4. Tweed C. Clinical Orthodontics. 1966, St Louis: Mosby.
5. Begg P R. Stone age man's dentition. Am J Orthod 1954; **40:** 298-312.
6. Little R M, Riedel R A, Stein A. Mandibular arch length increase during the mixed dentition: postretention evaluation of stability and relapse. Am J Orthod Dentofac Orthop 1990; **97:** 393-404.
7. Betteridge M A. The effects of interdental stripping on the labial segments evaluated one year out of retention. Br J Orthod 1981; **8:** 193-197.
8. Little R M. Stability and relapse of dental arch alignment. Br J Orthod 1990; **17:** 235-241.
9. Proffit W E. Forty-year review of extraction frequency at a university orthodontic clinic. Angle Orthod 1994; **64:** 407-414.
10. McCaul L K, Jenkins W M, Kay E J. The reasons for extraction of permanent teeth in Scotland: a 15-year follow-up study. Br Dent J 2001; **190:** 658-662.
11. Kirschen R H, O'Higgins E A, Lee R T. The Royal London Space Planning: an integration of space analysis and treatment planning: Part II: The effect of other treatment procedures on space. Am J Orthod Dentofacial Orthop 2000; **118:** 448-461.
12. Khurana M, Martin M V. Orthodontics and infective endocarditis. Br J Orthod 1999; **26:** 295-298.
13. Ericson S, Kurol J. Early treatment of palatally erupting maxillary canines by extraction of the primary canines. Eur J Orthod 1988; **10:** 283-295.
14. Bradbury A J. The influence of orthodontic extractions on the caries indices in schoolchildren in the United Kingdom. Comm Dent Health 1985; **2:** 75-82.
15. Canut J A. Mandibular incisor extraction: indications and long-term evaluation. Eur J Orthod 1986; **18:** 485-489.
16. Graber T M. New horizons in case analysis: clinical cephalometrics. Am J Orthod 1956; **53:** 439-454.
17. Tuverson D L. Anterior interocclusal relations. Part II. Am J Orthod 1980; **78:** 371-393.
18. Berg R, Gebauer U. Spontaneous changes in the mandibular arch following first premolar extractions. Eur J Orthod 1982; **4:** 93-98.
19. Vastardis H. The genetics of human tooth agenesis: new discoveries for understanding dental anomalies. Am J Orthod Dentofac Orthop 2000; **117:** 650-656.
20. Sandler P J, Atkinson R, Murray A M. For four sixes. Am J Orthod Dentofac Orthop 2000; **117:** 418-434.
21. Thomas P, Sandy J R. Should second molars be extracted? Dent Update 1995; **22:** 150-156.
22. National Clinical Guidelines. The management of patients with impacted third molar (syn. Wisdom) teeth. Royal College of Surgeons of England 1997.
23. Richardson M E, Richardson A. The effect of extraction of four second permanent molars on the incisor overbite. Eur J Orthod 1993; **15:** 291-296.
24. Schwarze C W. The influence of third molar germectomy - a comparative long term study. Abstract of Third International Congress, London 1973; 551-562.

IN BRIEF

- Anchorage is the resistance to unwanted tooth movement
- It can be obtained from a number of different sources
- Loss of anchorage can have a detrimental effect on treatment
- Safety is of prime importance when using extra-oral devices

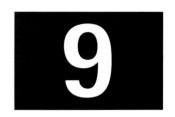

Anchorage control and distal movement

D. Roberts-Harry and J. Sandy

Anchorage is an important consideration when planning orthodontic tooth movement. Unwanted tooth movement known as loss of anchorage can have a detrimental effect on the treatment outcome. Anchorage can be sourced from the teeth, the oral mucosa and underlying bone, implants and extra orally. If extra-oral anchorage is used, particularly with a facebow then the use of at least two safety devices is mandatory.

Anchorage is defined as the resistance to unwanted tooth movement. Newton's third law states that every action has an equal and opposite reaction. This principle also applies to moving teeth. For example, if an upper canine is being retracted, the force applied to the tooth must be resisted by an equal and opposite force in the other direction. This equal and opposite force is known as anchorage.

Anchorage may be considered similar to a tug of war. Two equal sized people will pull each other together by an equal amount. Conversely a big person will generally pull a small one without being moved. However, if two or more smaller people combine then their chances of pulling a big person will increase. Similarly, the more teeth that are incorporated into an anchorage block, the more likely it is that desirable as opposed to undesirable tooth movements will occur. Undesirable movement of the anchor teeth is called loss of anchorage.

If an upper canine is to be retracted, with bodily movement using a fixed appliance, the force applied to the tooth will be approximately 100 g (Fig. 1a). Forces in the opposite direction varying from 67 g on the first permanent molar to 33 g on the upper second premolar resist this. Low levels will produce negligible tooth movement and the effect of a light force of 100 g would be to retract the canine with minimal anterior unwanted movement of the anchored teeth. However, if the force level is increased to say 300 g (Fig. 1b), the force levels on the anchor teeth increase dramatically to the level where unwanted tooth movements will occur. Although the canine may move a little distally,

the buccal teeth will also move mesially. Space for the canine retraction may be eliminated with insufficient space left for alignment of the anterior teeth. Figure 1c compares the root area of some of the upper teeth. The combined root area of the upper incisors and upper canines is around the same as that of the first molar and premolars. Therefore, if the upper labial segment including the upper canines is retracted in a block, there will be an equivalent mesial movement of the upper molar and upper premolar. These factors need to be very carefully considered in planning anchorage requirements and tooth movement.

Anchorage may be derived from four sources:

- Teeth
- Oral mucosa and underlying bone
- Implants
- Extra oral

TEETH

The anchorage supplied by the teeth can come from within the same arch as the teeth that are being moved (intra maxillary) or from the opposing arch (inter maxillary).

Intra maxillary anchorage

The anchorage provided by teeth depends on the size of the teeth, ie the root area of the teeth. Fig. 1c shows the root surface area of each of the teeth in the upper arch. The more teeth that are incorporated into an anchorage block the less likely unwanted tooth movement will occur. If a removable appliance is used, the base plate and retaining cribs should contact as many of

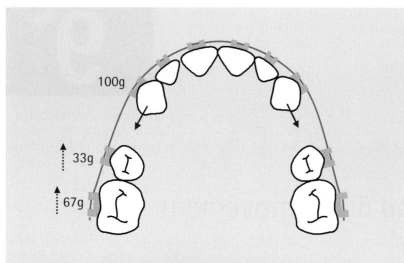

Fig. 1a A distalising force on the upper canine will produce a reciprocal force in the opposite direction on the anchor teeth. Provided the force level for bodily movement is kept low at about 100g then there will be minimal mesial movement of the anchor teeth

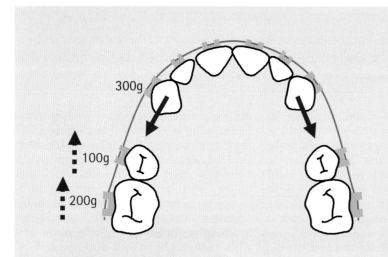

Fig. 1b As the distalising force level increases the reciprocal forces also increase with a greater risk of loss of anchorage

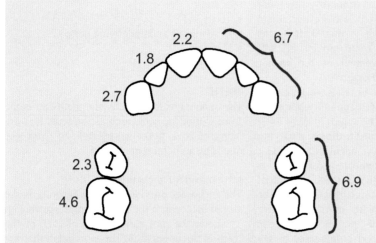

Fig. 1c The combined root surface area of the anterior teeth is almost the same as the molar and premolar. Attempting to move all the anterior teeth distally simultaneously will result in an equal mesial movement of the posterior teeth

the teeth as possible. Figure 2 illustrates the point. If upper canines are to be retracted with a removable appliance, cribs on the first permanent molars and upper incisors will not only help with retention but also increase the anchorage considerably. In addition, the base plate must contact the mesial surface of the upper second premolars and palatal to the upper incisors. If fixed appliances are to be used, the more teeth that are bracketed or banded, the greater will be the anchorage resistance (Fig. 3).

Inter maxillary anchorage

Teeth in the opposite arch can provide very useful and important sites of anchorage control as Figs 4a,b illustrate. Good inter-digitation of the buccal teeth can help prevent mesial movement of the buccal segment. Although there is only anecdotal evidence to support this view, many clinicians feel this can be a useful source of anchorage.

The second way that opposing teeth can be used is by means of elastics or springs running from one arch to the other. Class II elastics (Fig. 4c) run from the lower molars to the upper incisor region, whereas Class III elastics (Fig. 4d) run from the upper molars to the lower incisor region.

Inter-maxillary elastic are invaluable in many cases but do rely very heavily on good patient co-operation. The elastics need to be changed every day and if they break (which they frequently do) they must be replaced immediately. Class II elastics also will tend to have unwanted effects on the occlusion. They tend to tip the lower molars mesially and roll them lingually. In addition, they can produce extrusion of the upper labial segment and the lower molars. Whilst extrusion of the lower molars can help with overbite reduction, extrusion of the upper incisors is usually an unwanted side effect and has to be counteracted by adding an upward curve to the upper arch-wire known as an increased curve of Spee. Extrusion of the buccal teeth is undesirable in patients with increased lower face height and therefore Class II elastics should be used sparingly in these cases. Similarly Class III elastics can extrude the upper molars, tip them mesially and roll them palatally. Molar extrusion will decrease the overbite, which is usually undesirable in Class III cases. Elastics also tend to cant the occlusal plane and have been implicated in root resorption in the upper labial segment particularly if they are used for prolonged periods.

Functional appliances are another source of intermaxillary anchorage. Whilst some clinicians may believe these devices simply make the mandible grow, this is not the case and whatever mandibular growth does take place, is accompanied by quite substantial movement of the dentition over the apical base. This means that mesial tipping of the lower and distal tipping of the upper teeth occurs.

ORAL MUCOSA AND UNDERLYING BONE

Contact between the appliance and the labial or lingual mucosa can increase anchorage considerably for either fixed or removable appliances. Contact between an orthodontic appliance and the vault of the palate provides resistance to mesial movement of the posterior teeth. The anchorage provided by this means is considerably greater if there is a high vaulted palate as shown in Figure 5a, which will produce a greater buttressing effect. A shallow vaulted palate (Fig. 5b) will provide much less anchorage control because the appliance will simply tend to slide down the inclined plane of the palate.

The mucosa and underlying bone can also be used when fixed appliances are used, for example a Nance palatal arch (Fig. 5c). This is an acrylic button that lies on the most vertical part of the palate behind the upper incisors and is added to a trans-palatal arch. These buttons are again of more limited use if the palatal vault is shallow.

IMPLANTS

Osseo-integrated implants can be used as a very secure source of anchorage. Implants integrate with bone and do not have a periodontal membrane. Because of this they do not move when a force is applied to them and in some cases they can provide an ideal source of anchorage. Recently small implants for orthodontic use have been specifically designed and can be used in the retro-molar region to move teeth distally or anteriorly for mesial movement. Short 4mm implants can be

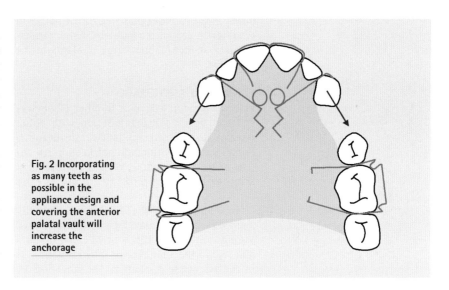

Fig. 2 Incorporating as many teeth as possible in the appliance design and covering the anterior palatal vault will increase the anchorage

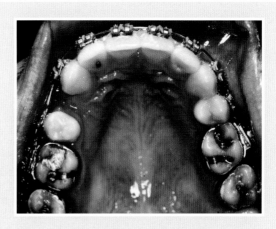

Fig. 3 When fixed appliances are used, as many teeth as possible are banded to increase the anchorage

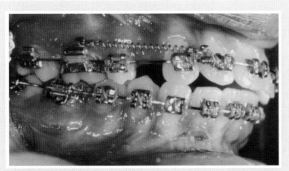

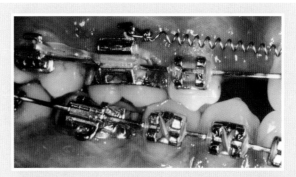

Fig. 4a,b Inter-digitation of the buccal occlusion can help increase anchorage

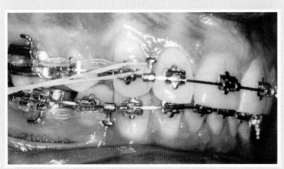

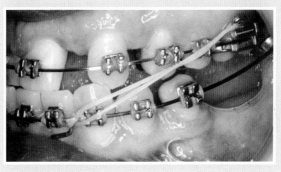

Fig. 4c Intermaxillary elastics use teeth in the opposite arch as a source of anchorage. Class II traction is shown here

Fig. 4d Class III elastics

paced in the anterior mid-line of the palate in the thickest part of the nasal crest and a trans-palatal bar then connects the implants to the teeth (Fig. 6).

EXTRA-ORAL ANCHORAGE

This can be applied via a number of devices and can be used in conjunction with either removable or fixed appliances. Headgear is not a recent invention and has been in use for over a century. Figure 7a is a picture of a Kingsley headgear, which was in use as early as 1861.

The force from the headgear is usually applied to the teeth via a face-bow (Klöen bow) as shown in Fig. 7b. This is fitted either to tubes attached to the appliance or integral with it as in the *en masse* appliance. The direction by which the force is applied can be varied depending on the type of headgear that is fitted. Headgear can be applied to both the maxillary and mandibular dentition, and there are a number of variations:

- Cervical
- Occipital
- Variable
- Reverse

Cervical Headgear

This is applied via an elastic strap or spring, which runs around the neck (Fig. 8a). It has the advantage of being relatively unobtrusive and easy to fit. However, it does tend to extrude the upper molars and tip them distally because of the downward and backward direction of force. This later effect can be counteracted to some degree by adjusting the height and length of the outer bow. Cervical headgear should not be attached to removable appliances because it is prone to dislodge the appliance and propel it to the back of the mouth.

Occipital

This is also known as high pull headgear and is applied via an occipitally placed head-cap (Fig. 8b). It is easy to fit but is more obvious than the neck strap and tends to roll off the head unless carefully adjusted. Because the force is in a more upward direction, there is generally less distal tipping of the upper molar and less extrusion, but also less distal movement than with cervical headgear. The tipping and extrusion effect again depend on the length and height of the outer bow.

Variable

This applies a force part way between cervical and occipital (Fig. 8c) and is our preferred choice. It takes slightly longer to fit than either cervical or occipital and is more obtrusive. However it is secure and comfortable and the vector of the force can be varied to produce relatively less tipping and/or extrusion.

Whilst headgear is a very useful source of anchorage, it has a number of disadvantages. These are as follows:

- Safety
- Clinical time
- Compliance
- Operator preference

The most important of these problems is the fact that headgear can be dangerous and a number of facial and serious eye injuries have been reported in the literature.[1-3] The Standards and Safety Committee of the British Orthodontic Society (BOS) have addressed these concerns. An advice sheet produced by the BOS is essential reading for anyone who wishes to use headgear.[4]

The main problems with headgear safety relate to the prongs at the end of the face-bow that fit into the headgear tubes on the intra-oral appliance. It is possible for the bow to become dislodged, either because it is pulled out of the mouth or when the patient rolls over when they are asleep. The recoil effect from the elastics can damage the teeth, oral mucosa, soft tissues of the face and most seriously, the eyes. In order to minimise these problem various safety devices have been suggested. These involve re-curving the distal end of the wire, using plastic coated face bows and various locking springs.[5,6] In addition a variety of snap-away face bows have been produced. If these are pulled beyond a pre set distance, the neck strap comes apart and prevents any recoil injury. Another popular method of preventing recoil is to fit a rigid safety strap, which prevents the bow from coming out of the mouth if it disengages from the tubes. Some examples of these safety devices are shown in Figures 8a-i.

The importance of headgear safety cannot be over emphasized and it is recommended that two safety mechanisms are simultaneously used, for example a locking spring and a snap away headgear or a safety face-bow and rigid safety strap.

Reverse

Reverse or protraction headgear is useful for mesial movement of the teeth, either to close spaces or help to correct a reverse overjet. It does not employ a face-bow, which is an advantage but instead employs intra-oral hooks to which elastics are applied (Fig. 9a,b).

LOSS OF ANCHORAGE

This is defined as the unplanned and unexpected movement of the anchor teeth during orthodontic treatment.

There are several causes of loss of anchorage. Some examples of these are:

- Poor appliance design
- Poor appliance adjustment
- Poor patient wear

Poor appliance design

Failure to adequately retain the appliance, or incorporate as many teeth into the anchor block as possible are common causes of anchorage loss. If fixed appliances are used, as many

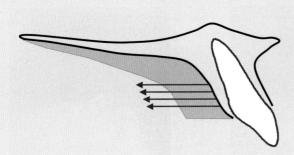

Fig. 5a A steep anterior palatal vault is a useful source of anchorage due to the buttressing effect

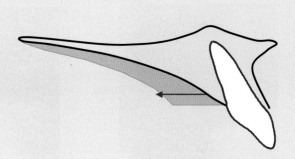

Fig. 5b A shallow palatal vault provides less anchorage

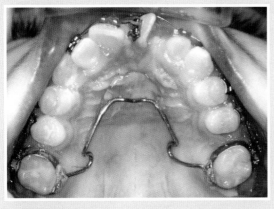

Fig. 5c The palatal vault can be used for removable or fixed appliances. An example of a Nance button is shown here

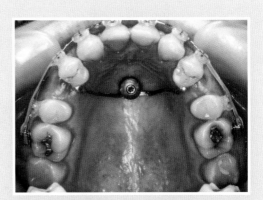

Fig. 6 An osseo-integrated implant with a bonded palatal arch is being used to help close space in the upper arch without retroclining the upper incisors

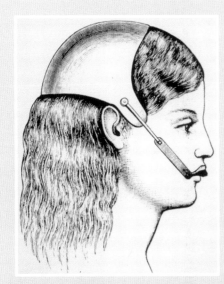

Fig. 7a An early Kingsley headgear circa 1860

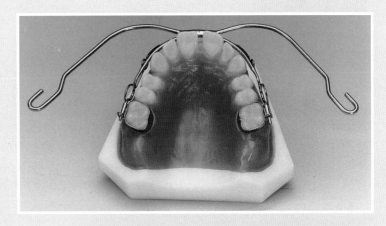

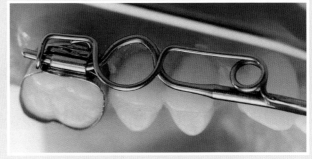

Fig. 7b,c A facebow (Klöen bow) is attached to tubes welded to bands on the molars

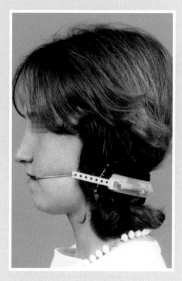

Fig. 8a A neck strap. Note the snap away safety mechanism

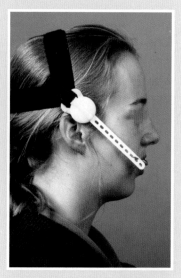

Fig. 8b An occipital (high pull) headgear again with a snap away safety system

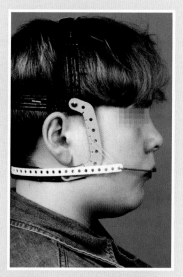

Fig. 8c A variable pull Interlandii headgear. A rigid plastic strip is employed as a safety mechanism to prevent the facebow disengaging from the molar bands and coming out of the mouth

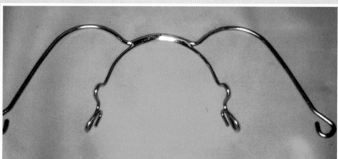
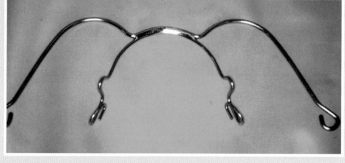

Fig. 8d,e The end of the facebow can be re-curved to improve safety

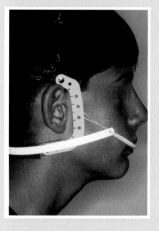
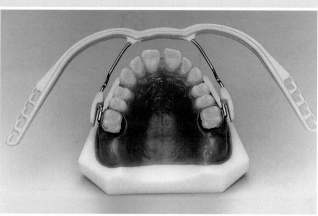

Fig. 8f,g A plastic coated facebow together with a safety neck-strap

Fig. 8h,i A Samuels locking spring. This secures the face bow preventing accidental disengagement. This should be used in conjunction with a safety neck strap or snap away headgear

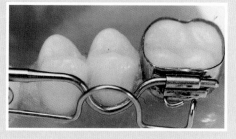
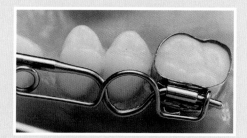

anchor teeth as possible should be banded in order to produce optimum anchorage. Removable appliances should have adequate retention using appropriate well-adjusted cribs or clasps with as much contact with the teeth and oral mucosa as possible.

Poor appliance adjustment

The use of excessive force or trying to move too many teeth at the same time may result in unwanted movement of the anchor teeth. To avoid loss of anchorage, simultaneous multiple teeth movement should be avoided. If the appliance is poorly adjusted so that it doesn't fit very well, or the force levels applied to the teeth are too high, then undesired tooth movement may occur. High force levels produced by over activation are one of the key reasons for anchorage loss.

The optimal force for movement of a single rooted tooth is about 25–40 g for tipping and about 75 g for bodily movement. If the force is too low there will be very little movement, whereas too much force may result in loss of anchorage. Excess force does not increase the rate of tooth retraction as illustrated in Fig. 10.[7] As the force levels rise the rate of tooth tipping also increases up to about 40 g. Beyond this very little extra tooth movement occurs. Thus increasing the force levels above about 40 g will not increase the rate of tooth tipping.

The force levels that wires from fixed or removable appliances exert on teeth usually depends on the following:

- The material the wire is made from
- The amount it is deflected
- The length of the wire
- The thickness of the wire

Steel wire will exert a force that is directly proportional to the amount the wire is deflected up to its elastic limit. Figure 11 demonstrates how decreasing the wire thickness and increasing the length (sometimes by adding loops) controls the force produced.

Modern alloys such as super elastic nickel titanium wires do not act in the same way as steel. These remarkable wires are capable of producing

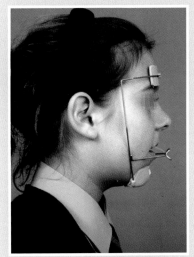
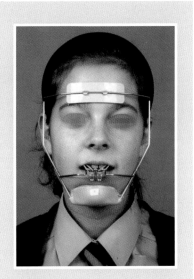

Fig. 9a, b A reverse, or protraction headgear

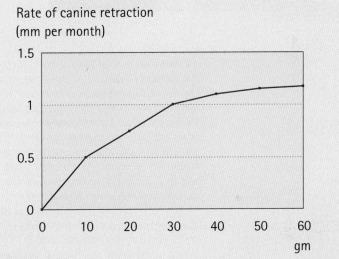

Rate of canine retraction (mm per month)

Fig. 10 The graph shows how increased force levels do not necessarily increase the rate of tooth movement. The y axis shows the rate of movement in mm. The x axis is the amount of tipping force applied to the tooth. As the force level initially rises the rate of tooth movement also increases. Above about 40 g the rate slows down and very little additional tooth movement occurs. There will however be a greater risk of loss of anchorage with increased force levels

Fig. 11 A 0.5 mm diameter wire can be deflected more than a 0.6 mm wire without increasing the force level. Thus a greater degree of activation is possible and the appliance will require less frequent adjustments. Similarly increasing the length of the wire, for example by incorporating loops allows a greater degree of wire deflection. The force characteristics may also be changed by altering the material the wire is made from

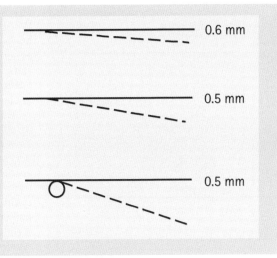

0.6 mm

0.5 mm

0.5 mm

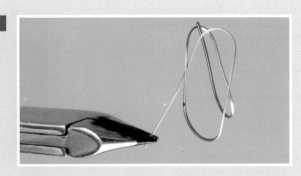

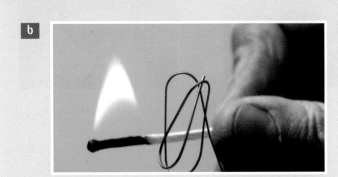

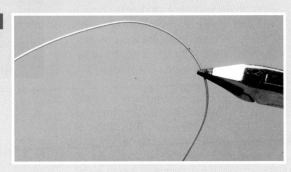

Fig. 12a–c Super elastic heat activated wires produce a light continuous force almost regardless of the amount of deflection. When cooled they become very flexible (12a) but return to their original shape as they warm in the mouth (12b,c)

a continuous level of force almost independent of the amount of deflection and have transformed the use of fixed appliances in recent years. Heat activated wire is now available that will increase its force level as the temperature changes. These wires exhibit a so-called shape memory effect. If the wire is cooled and tied into the teeth it deflects easily into position. As the wire warms in the mouth it gradually returns to its original shape moving the teeth with it (Figs12a–c).

For optimal tooth movement it is important that continuous gentle forces are applied to the teeth. Fixed appliances are ideal for doing this. When removable appliances are worn, the patient should wear them full-time except for cleaning and playing contact sports. Part-time wear produces intermittent forces on the teeth and is likely to reduce the rate of movement.

When a force is applied to a tooth, there is an initial period of movement as the periodontal membrane is compressed (Fig. 13). No tooth movement occurs for a few days after this, as cells are recruited in order to remodel the socket as well as the periodontal membrane. This cell recruitment takes a few days and is known as the lag effect. Part-time wear of appliances will not allow efficient cell recruitment and the lag phase will not be passed which may result in poor tooth movement. This is another reason why fixed appliances, which cannot be left out of the mouth by patients, are much more effective than removable appliances at achieving a satisfactory treatment outcome.

RETRIEVAL AND PRESERVATION OF ANCHORAGE

Extra-oral devices can be used for distal movement as well as anchorage reinforcement. For anchorage control wearing the headgear at night-time only is usually enough. In order to produce distal movement, the patient should wear the appliance in excess of 12 hours usually for the evenings as well as at nighttime. While some practitioners increase the force levels for distal movement purposes, it is our experience that this is not necessary and a force of approximately 250–300 g per side is adequate for both distal movement and anchorage control.

Many devices have been described to reduce or eliminate the need for headgear. These are however of limited use and can only produce a very small amount of extra space. If these gadgets are used without anchorage re-enforcement unwanted mesial movement of the anchor teeth could occur. Figures 14a–c shows one example known as a Jones jig. To produce distal movement of the molars the anchorage is reinforced with an anterior trans-palatal arch. A jig incor-

Fig. 13 Tooth movement requires light continuous forces. In this graph tooth movement in mm is shown on the y-axis and time in days on the x-axis. If a force is applied to a tooth the periodontal membrane is compressed and there is a small amount of initial movement. Movement then stops as bone cells are recruited and the socket starts to be remodeled. After about 14 days sufficient recruitment and remodeling has occurred to allow the tooth to move

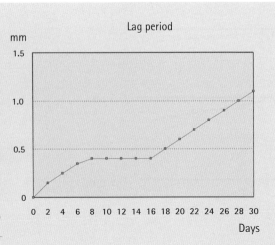

Fig. 14a–c A Jones jig for distal movement of the molars (14a). A palatal arch is fitted to the first premolars to increase the anterior anchorage. A jig is then inserted into the buccal arch wire and headgear tubes. An open nickel titanium coil spring is then slid over the shaft of the jig and compressed by sliding a collar onto the shaft and tying it to the premolar (14b). This then uses the upper premolars and palatal vault to distalise the molars (14c). Note the simultaneous mesial movement of the first premolars which is a sign of anchorage loss

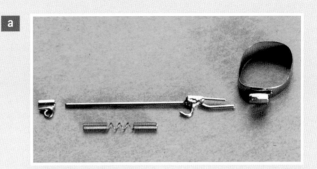

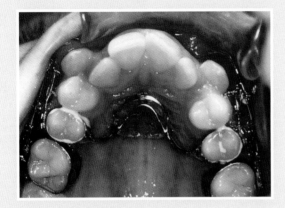

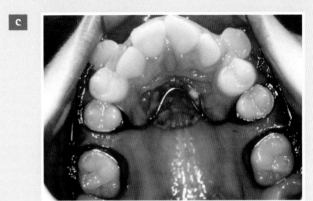

porating a nickel-titanium coil spring is inserted into molar tubes and tied into the premolar bands. The molars are distalised using the anterior teeth from premolar to premolar as the anchorage block. It is important to note the loss of anchorage that is occurring as demonstrated by the simultaneous mesial movement of the first premolars. Once distal movement of the molars has been achieved the anchorage reinforcement can be transferred to the molars (palatal arch or Nance button) and the premolars, canines and incisors retracted. True anchorage re-enforcement with these devices is difficult to achieve and headgear, or implants must still be considered the mainstay of producing effective distal movement.

Thanks to Mr. R Cousley for figure 6 and Mr. J Kinelan for figures 14a–c

1. Booth-Mason S, Birnie D. Penetrating eye injury from orthodontic headgear. *Eur J Orthod* 1998; **10:** 111-114.
2. Samuels R H A, M Willner F, Knox J, Jones M L. A national survey of orthodontic face bow injuries in the YUK and Eire. *Br J Orthod* 1996; **23:** 11-20.
3. Samuels R H A, Jones M L. Orthodontic face bow injuries and safety equipment. *Eur J Orthod* 1994; **16:** 385-394.
4. British Orthodontic Society, 291 Grays Inn Road, London WC1X 8QJ.
5. Postlethwaite K. The range and effectiveness of safety headgear products. *Eur J Orthod* 1988; **11:** 228-234.
6. Samuels R H A, Evans S M, Wigglesworth S W. Safety catch for Kloen face bow. *J Clin Orthod* 1993; **27:** 138-141.
7. Crabb J J, Wilson H J. The relation between orthodontic spring force and space closure. *Dent Pract Dent Res* 1972; **22:** 233-240.

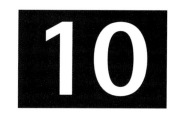
IN BRIEF

- Check all 10-year-olds for the position of their permanent canines by initial clinical examination and palpation, if necessary with further radiographs to locate possible impactions
- Check for late eruption of permanent incisors, if one incisor has erupted, the others should not be far behind. If the permanent lateral incisors have erupted but not the permanent central incisors then suspicion of impaction should be heightened
- Refer too early rather than too late

Impacted teeth

D. Roberts-Harry and J. Sandy

This section deals with the important issue of impacted teeth. Impacted canines in Class I uncrowded cases can be improved by removal of the deciduous canines. There is some evidence that this is true for both buccal and palatal impactions. Treatment of impacted canines is lengthy and potentially hazardous. Interceptive measures are effective and preferred to active treatment. Supernumerary teeth may also cause impaction of permanent incisors, their early diagnosis and appropriate treatment is essential to optimise final outcomes. If there are any doubts about impacted teeth it is better to refer too early than too late, this latter option may unnecessarily extend the length of treatment as well as the treatment required.

This section brings together the information general dental practitioners need in order to diagnose and deal effectively with impacted teeth.

IMPACTED CANINES

A canine that is prevented from erupting into a normal position, either by bone, tooth or fibrous tissue, can be described as impacted. Impacted maxillary canines are seen in about 3% of the population. The majority of impacted canines are palatal (85%), the remaining 15% are usually buccal. There is sex bias, 70% occur in females. One of the biggest dangers is that they can cause resorption of the roots of the lateral or central incisors and this is seen in about 12% of the cases.

The cause of impaction is not known, but these teeth develop at the orbital rims and have a long path of eruption before they find their way into the line of the arch. Consequently in crowded cases there may be insufficient room for them in the arch and they may be deflected. It seems that the root of the lateral incisor is important in the guidance of upper permanent canines to their final position. There is also some evidence that there may be genetic input into the aetiology of the impaction.

Late referral or misdiagnosis of impacted canines places a significant burden on the patient in relation to how much treatment they will subsequently need. If the canines are in poor positions it will require a considerable amount of treatment and effort in order to get them into the line of the arch and a judgement must be made as to whether it is worth it. Sacrificing the canine is unsatisfactory since this presents a challenge to the restorative dentist, an aesthetic problem and by definition, cannot be used to guide the occlusion. There are times when it might be sensible to consider its loss, but early diagnosis can make a significant difference to how much treatment is needed by the patient.

DIAGNOSIS

It is easy to miss non-eruption of the permanent canines, but there are some markers which should increase suspicion of possible impaction. Any case with a deep bite, missing lateral incisors or peg-shaped upper lateral incisors needs a detailed examination. Figure 1 shows such a case and in this instance both canines were significantly impacted on the palatal aspect. The retained deciduous canine is self evident. Other clues include root and crown positions. Figure 2 shows a lateral incisor which is proclined. There

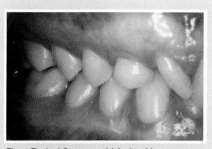

Fig. 1 Typical features which should arouse suspicion of impacted canines. There is a deep bite and a small peg-shaped lateral incisor. The retained deciduous canine is obvious. In this patient both upper permanent canines were palatally positioned

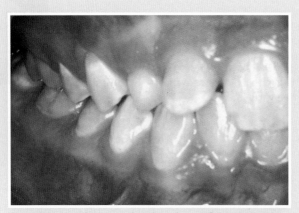

Fig. 2 There are clues as to the whereabouts of the upper right permanent canine in this patient. The upper right lateral crown is proclined because the upper right permanent canine is buccally positioned and therefore places pressure on the root moving the crown of the lateral incisor labially and the root of the lateral incisor palatally

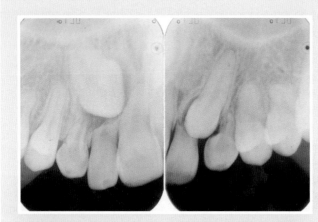

Fig. 3 Consequences of failure to diagnose impacted canines. This radiograph shows the roots of the upper lateral incisor to be resorbing

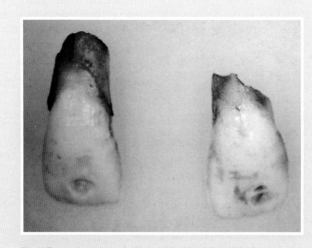

Fig. 4 The patient shown in Figure 3 had both lateral incisors removed because of the severe root resorption caused by the unerupted permanent canines

is a retained deciduous canine and the permanent canine lies buccal which moves the root of the lateral incisor palatally and the crown labially.

Any general dental examination of a patient from the age of 10 years should include palpation for the permanent canine on the buccal aspect. It is possible to locate the canines with palpation, but this will lead to some false observations. For instance, the buccal root of a decidous canine, if it is not resorbing, can feel like the crown of the permanent tooth. It is therefore important to back up clinical examination with radiographs. Failure to make these observations will eventually result in patients complaining of loose incisors; inevitably some permanent canines will resorb adjacent teeth with devastating efficiency as shown in Figures 3 and 4.

WHAT ARE THE BEST RADIOGRAPHIC VIEWS TO LOCATE CANINES?

Most patients undergoing routine orthodontic screening will have a dental pantomogram. Location of tooth position requires two radiographs in different positions. In the interests of radiation hygiene it is sensible to use this as a base x-ray and to take further location radiographs in relation to the dental pantomogram. An anterior occlusal radiograph allows this and the principle of vertical parallax can be used to locate the position of the canine. The tube has to shift in order to take an anterior occlusal and it moves in a vertical direction. If the tooth crown appears to move in the direction of the tube shift (ie vertically) then the tooth will be positioned on the palatal aspect. If the crown appears to move in the opposite direction it is buccal and if it shows no movement at all it is in the line of the arch (Figures 5 to 7). This also provides a reasonably detailed intra-oral view in cases of root resorption.

Although there are other radiographic techniques which can be used to locate canines, this method works well. If there are difficulties in being sure of the exact location then two periapicals taken of the region with a horizontal shift of the tube may give slightly better precision. The periapical radiographs will also give good detail of the roots of adjacent teeth, particularly the lateral incisors. The proximity of the canine crown to incisor roots does make them vulnerable to root resorption. The percentage of teeth adjacent to the crown of the canine which undergo some form of resorption is probably quite high at the microscopic level. No extractions should be contemplated until the canines have been located. Figure 8 shows a dental pantomogram of a patient who had both upper and lower first premolars removed as part of a treatment plan, but where the canines had not been located beforehand. The dental pantomogram clearly shows the poor position of the canines and subsequent treatment involved the removal of the permanent canines since their position was deemed hopeless and movement of the canines may well have resulted in root resorp-

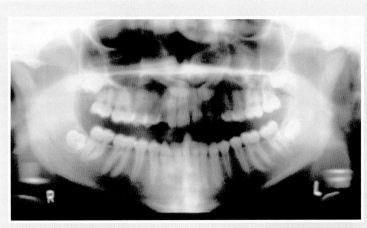

Fig. 5 Orthopantomograph of patient where the two canines are clearly impacted

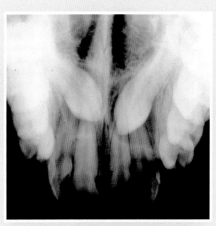

Fig. 6 Anterior occlusal radiograph of the same patient shown in Figure 5. Both canines are now more apically positioned and therefore these teeth have moved with the tube shift and are palatally positioned

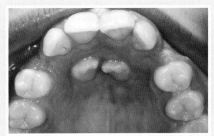

Fig. 7 Same patient as in Figures 5 and 6 with both permanent canines exposed surgically and on the palatal aspect

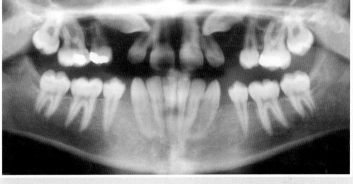

Fig. 8 Dental pantomogram of a patient who had had all four first premolars removed without sufficient diagnostic information. The upper permanent canines are in a very poor position and with the distinct possibility of some root resorption it was felt that the upper permanent canines should be removed and replaced prosthetically

tion of the incisors. The canines had to be replaced prosthetically and it would be difficult to see how a legal defence of this situation could be raised.

INTERCEPTIVE MEASURES FOR CANINES
One of the most significant publications in the orthodontic literature came from Ericson & Kurol (1988)[1] who demonstrated that extraction of upper deciduous canines where the upper permanent canines were developing on the palatal aspect, resulted in nearly an 80% chance of correcting the impaction. The paper was very specific about what types of malocclusions this could be applied to. Nearly all the cases were Class I with no incisor crowding. This is important to emphasise, a subsequent follow-up paper[2] confirmed their original observation and also indicated that the technique could not be applied easily to crowded cases and in some cases this would result in a worsening of the situation rather than an improvement. The dental pantomogram of a patient is shown in Figure 9. The canines are palatally positioned. Since this was an uncrowded case, the deciduous canines were extracted and Figure 10 shows that both the

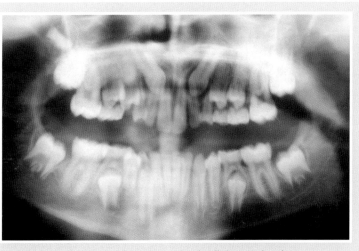

Fig. 9 Dental pantomogram of a patient with palatally impacted canines

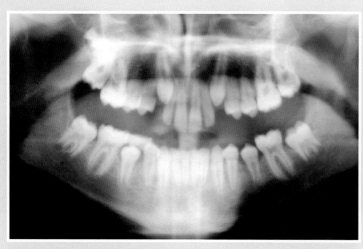

Fig. 10 The same patient as in Figure 9. The dental pantomogram clearly shows that both canines have disimpacted and are now erupting in the line of the arch. The only active treatment was extraction of both upper deciduous canines

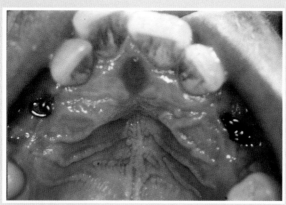

Fig. 11 Palatally impacted canines which have had a flap raised and gold chain bonded to the crowns of the permanent canines

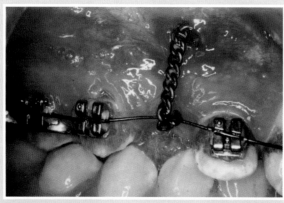

Fig. 12 A bucally positioned canine has had a gold chain attached but in an incorrect position. The chain should exit mid alveolus and from keratinised mucosa

permanent canines erupted with no orthodontic assistance. Clearly this saved the patient a considerable amount of treatment and early appropriate referral would be wise if a general dental practitioner is unsure. The interceptive measure of extracting deciduous canines works well if carried out between the ages of 11–13 years. The closer the crowns are to the mid-line the worse the prognosis. It is worth re-emphasising that this works best in Class I uncrowded cases.

TREATMENT OF CANINES

The treatment of buccally or palatally impacted canines involves exposure and then a form of traction to pull the tooth into the correct position in the arch. Palatally impacted teeth can be exposed and allowed to erupt. This tends to form a better gingival attachment since the tooth is erupting into attached mucosa. This cuff may be lost on the palatal aspect as the tooth is brought into line. Some operators prefer to raise a flap, attach a bracket pad with a gold chain to the tooth in theatre and then replace the flap. Traction is subsequently applied to the chain and the tooth pulled through the mucosa (Fig. 11). There is some evidence that this procedure is less successful than a straight forward exposure. It also has a disadvantage that if the bonded attachment fails then a further operation, either to expose or reattach, is needed. The advantage with this technique is that the root usually needs less buccal torque once the crown is in position.

If the canine is moderately high and buccal, it will not be possible to expose the tooth since it will then erupt through unattached mucosa and an apically repositioned flap should be considered. If it is very high, it is not possible to apically reposition the flap and therefore it is better in this situation to raise a flap and bond an attachment with a gold chain. It is critical that the chain passes underneath the attached mucosa and exits in the space where the permanent canine will eventually be placed as in Figure 11. If it is not placed in this situation and exits out of non-keratinised mucosa the final gingival attachment will be poor (Fig. 12).

Other options include:

Accept and observe
Leaving the deciduous canine in place and either observing the impacted canine or removing it. Long term, the deciduous canine will need prosthetic replacement.

Extract the impacted canine
If there is a good contact between the lateral incisor and the first premolar then it has to be carefully considered whether this should be accepted. The purists of occlusion will argue that the premolar is not capable of providing good canine guidance. Aesthetically there are problems since the palatal cusp hangs down. This can be disguised by grinding or rotating the tooth

orthodontically so that the palatal cusp is positioned more distally. The placement of a veneer on the premolar is another way of improving the appearance.

Transplantation

Canine transplantation has received poor press in the past. Many of the problems arose because the canines were transplanted with a closed apex. These teeth were seldom followed up with root fillings on the basis that they would revascularise. This is unlikely through a closed apex and it is preferable to treat them as if they were non-vital. Transplantation is an option which should only be reserved for teeth that are in almost an impossible position and where there is extensive hypodontia or other tooth loss.

Implants

Implants are also an option and as single tooth implants improve, this may become more favoured in future. It is important to remember that implants in a growing child will ankylose and appear to submerge as the alveolus continues to develop. These are not therefore an option until the patient is at least 20 years of age.

Correction of canine position
Favourable indications for correction of impacted canines.

Canines are moved most easily into their correct position if the root apex is in a favourable position. If the tooth lies horizontally it is extremely difficult to correct this and generally the closer the tooth to the midline the more difficult the correction will be. Treatment is nearly always lengthy and can damage adjacent teeth. Figure 13 shows a lateral incisor adjacent to a palatally impacted canine where the opposite reaction to

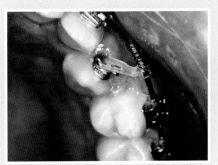

Fig. 14 Palatally positioned canine being moved with power chain into the correct position

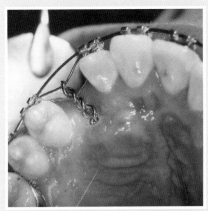

Fig. 15 A 'piggy back' flexible wire has been deflected in order to apply traction to the gold chain which has been attached to a palatally positioned canine. There is a stiff base wire which prevents unwanted reactions to this traction

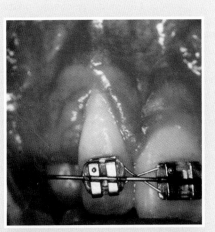

Fig. 13 A lateral incisor adjacent to a palatally impacted canine. When the canine is pulled labially the reaction will be for the lateral root to move labially. It is essential therefore to use thick rectangular wires during the movement of palatally positioned canines. Further labial movement of the lateral root would be potentially damaging to the periodontal attachment

pulling the palatal canine out is the labial positioning of the lateral incisor root. Obviously this is not favourable and the gingival recession will worsen. The force to move the canines can be obtained from elastomeric chain or thread. Figure 14 shows elastomeric chain being used to pull the canine labially. An attachment has been bonded to the tooth, but as the tooth moves to its correct position it will be necessary to rebond it. Moving the tooth over the bite sometimes requires the occlusion to be disengaged with a bite plane or glass ionomer cement build ups on posterior teeth, for a few weeks.

An alternative is to use a smaller diameter nickel titanium 'piggy back' wire with a stiff base wire to align the tooth (Fig. 15). The thicker base wire maintains the archform by resisting local distortion caused by the traction on the canine. The nickel titanium piggy back wire produces flexibility and a constant low force, unlike elastomeric chain or thread which have a high initial force and then a rapid decay of this force. It is better not to tie the piggy back in fully as the wire needs to be able to slide distally as the canine moves labially. If tied in fully the friction does not allow this function. It also helps if the

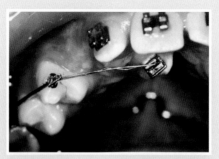

Fig. 16 Beta titanium sectional arch which is both formable and flexible can be deflected to apply traction to move the impacted canine buccally

piggy back wires run through auxiliary tubes on the first molar bands. One further method which has gained some popularity is the use of a sectional archwire made of beta-titanium alloy. This wire is formable and flexible, it can be deflected as a sectional arm and pulls the canine labially. It is important to use a palatal arch which cross braces the molars to prevent them moving into crossbite as an opposite force reaction to the buccal movement of the canines (Fig. 16).

The use of heat activated nickel titanium alloys has also done much to improve the efficiency of moving impacted canines into the correct position. Figures 17 and 18 show a sequence of tooth movements where a nickel titanium alloy has been deflected, after cooling with a refrigerant, into the bracket. The length of time between the two slides was 8 weeks and

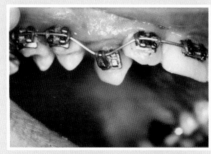

Fig. 17 The impacted canine has had a heat activated nickel titanium wire deflected into the bracket

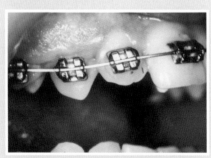

Fig. 18 Same patient as shown in Figure 17 nearly 8 weeks later where significant tooth movement has taken place

it can be seen how much tooth movement has occurred. The transpalatal arch is also useful anchorage for vertical and antero-posterior tooth movements.

WHAT CAN GO WRONG?

There are a number of problems with moving permanent canines from either a buccal or a palatal position. By and large, the older the patient the less chance there is of succeeding, and certainly moving canines in adults requires caution. If the canines have to be moved a considerable distance then ankylosis is a distinct possibility as well as loss of vascular supply and therefore pulp death. Treatment often takes in excess of 2 years and it is important to maintain a motivated and co-operative patient. It is necessary to create sufficient space for the canine to be aligned and this is usually around 9 mm.

The periodontal condition of canines that have been moved into the correct position in the arch can deteriorate, this is particularly true if care has not been taken to ensure that the canine either erupts or is positioned into keratinised mucosa. There may also be damage to adjacent teeth during surgery, or indeed the surgeons can damage the canine itself with burs or other instruments. Figure 19 shows the crown of a canine which has clearly been grooved by a bur which was used for bone removal when the canine was exposed. It is quite easy to induce root resorption of adjacent teeth (either the lateral incisor or the first premolar), particularly if care is not taken in the direction of traction applied to the impacted canine. Loss of blood supply of adjacent teeth can also occur. It is quite common at the end of treatment to see a slightly darker crown of the permanent canine, this probably results from either a change in vascularity and vitality of the canines, or potentially haemoglobin products can be produced and seep into the dentine thus changing the colour of the overlying enamel. The worst scenario of all is that the canine ankyloses and will not move. The protracted length of treatment also results in patients abandoning treatment.

Despite all of our improvements in treatment mechanics and diagnosis for impacted canines, the eruption path is often unpredictable. Canines which have a seemingly hopeless prog-

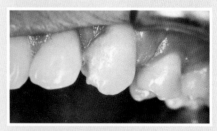

Fig. 19 The crown of this canine was grooved by a bur used during bone removal when the canine was exposed

nosis can sometimes correct their position and erupt. Nevertheless, to sit and observe a patient where the canines are clearly in difficulty without referral to a specialist would be difficult to defend legally. Hopefully the days of patients arriving in orthodontic departments with retained deciduous teeth at the age of 16 will diminish as the profession takes on the challenge of life long learning.

OTHER IMPACTED TEETH

The most common cause of unerupted maxillary incisors is the presence of a supernumerary tooth. These are often typed as follows:

- Conical
- Tuberculate
- Odontomes (complex or compound)
- Supplemental teeth

There are some conditions which have a genetic basis where impacted teeth are seen more frequently and this includes cleidocranial dysplasia, cleft lip and palate, gingival fibromatosis and Down's Syndrome.

It is worth remembering that most central incisors should have erupted by the age of 7 and lateral incisors by the age of 8. Surprisingly, most referrals for impacted maxillary incisors are when the patient is 9 years of age. This delay in diagnosis could potentially influence the outcome and it is important that when the contralateral incisor has erupted 6 months previously there is likely to be a problem. Similarly, if the lateral incisors erupt well before the central incisor then consideration should be given to investigating further (Fig. 20).

It is perfectly possible that a supernumerary tooth may be present and not affect the eruption of the incisors (Fig. 21). Indeed one of the clinical signs that a supernumerary may be present is the evidence of spacing where a supernumerary is in the midline and causing a diastema between the upper incisors. The different types of supernumerary teeth seem to have different implications for treatment.

Conical supernumerary teeth are small and peg-shaped, they usually have a root and they do not often affect incisor eruption (Fig. 21), but if they are in the midline they can cause a median diastema. They should only be removed if they are adjacent to incisors which need to undergo root movement. Potentially the movement of the root against the supernumerary tooth could cause resorption of an incisor root.

Where the supernumerary teeth are tuberculate these usually have no roots and develop palatally. They often prevent the eruption of central incisors and if they do, they need to be removed (Fig. 22). Complex and compound odontomes are rare, but can similarly prevent eruption of the permanent incisors and also need to be removed. Obviously, radiographs are needed to confirm any clinical observations about impacted teeth and parallax used in the same way as for canines in order to locate the position of the supernumerary teeth. Eighty per

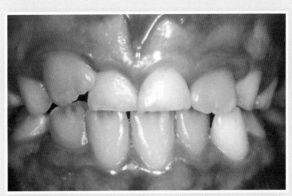

Fig. 20 This patient has both her lateral incisors fairly well erupted but retained deciduous teeth. This could easily have been diagnosed sooner and may influence the outcome of final tooth position

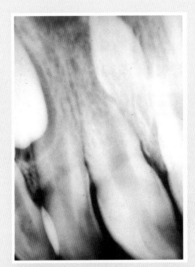

Fig. 21 Conical supernumerary which has not inhibited the eruption of the permanent incisors. The supernumerary is in the midline

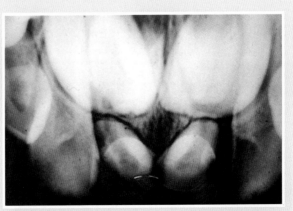

Fig. 22 Anterior occlusal radiograph which shows both upper lateral incisors to have erupted, both upper deciduous central incisors are retained and the upper permanent central incisors are unerupted. There are two tuberculate supernumeraries present which are associated with the non-eruption of these upper permanent central incisors

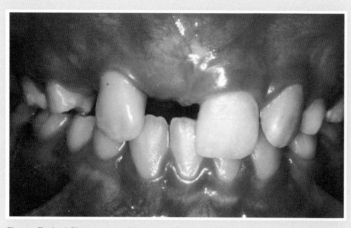

Fig. 23 Typical fibrous tissue impaction of the permanent incisor. In this patient a supernumerary had been removed 9 months earlier. The tooth will only require a small exposure on the palatal aspect to enable it to erupt. The bulge in the labial mucosa is clearly evident and this is where the crown will sit

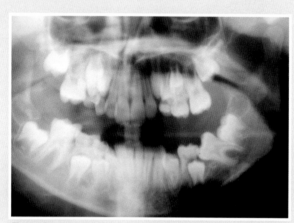

Fig. 24 Dental pantomogram of a patient who appears to have severe impaction of her lower left second premolar

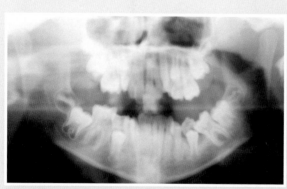

Fig. 25 This same patient as in Figure 24, 9 months later where there has been good eruption of the lower left second premolar. Eventually this tooth made its way fully into the line of the arch and it was possible to upright the lower left first molar

cent of supernumerary teeth occur in the anterior part of the maxilla and there is a male to female ratio of 2:1. The incidence in the population as a whole varies, but is somewhere in the region of 1–2%.

Treatment of impacted supernumeraries

Although guidelines have been published from the Royal College of Surgeons,[3] these review what the options are rather than defining what the best treatment is. In part this is due to a lack of good research to show what the best methods are.

Obviously if there is an obstruction the sooner it is removed the better. Some suggest exposing the incisor at the same time or attachment of a gold chain in order to prevent re-operation if the tooth fails to erupt. However, this is potentially damaging, particularly if bone has to be removed in order to expose or bond an attachment to the tooth with a gold chain brought out through the mucosa in order to place traction and move the impacted incisor.

If diagnosed early and the supernumerary is removed when the apex of the incisor is open then eruption of the tooth can be anticipated. Even if there is a need to re-operate at a later date, if the tooth has come further down it is much easier to either expose the tooth or raise a flap and place an attachment on an incisal edge that is now much closer to its correct position. Often incisors will erupt quite a long way and then become impacted in fibrous tissue (Fig. 23). In this situation it only requires a small exposure usually on the palatal aspect to allow the tooth to come down. Apically repositioned flaps are often disastrous and produce poor mucosal attachment. In the main they should be avoided.

Fixed appliances are usually needed in order to regain lost space where adjacent teeth have drifted and these appliances are also useful if traction does need to be applied to the impacted teeth. Removable appliances in this situation are often cumbersome, although they have been used with a magnet bonded to the unerupted tooth and a further magnet embedded into the removable appliance in order to bring the tooth down. The use of fixed appliances in this situation allows alignment, space management and overbite correction. Ultimately the early diagnosis of unerupted teeth is the biggest contribution a practitioner can make to the management of impacted teeth.

IMPACTED PREMOLARS

Where crowding exists or where there has been early loss of deciduous molars, premolars are sometimes unable to erupt. Often relief of crowding (usually extraction of first premolars) allows impacted second premolars to erupt. Second premolars do seem to have enormous potential to erupt and given time these teeth often find their way into the arch (Figs 24 and 25). Often in the upper arch they displace palatally. There may also be clues from the deciduous teeth. If the deciduous teeth become ankylosed they often appear to submerge as alveolar bone growth continues. This may indicate the absence of a second premolar, but sometimes this submergence can be seen when permanent successors are present. Most of these situations will resolve, but it is thought wise to consider removing the second deciduous molar if it slips below the contact points and there is then space loss as the molar tips forward. Where first molar mesial migration compromises the contact point relationship, space maintenance might be considered. Figure 26 shows a radiograph of a patient who appears to have generalised submergence since all second deciduous molars are seen to be submerging in all four quadrants. In this situation continued observation of the development of the occlusion with appropriate loss of deciduous molars is essential. With the extensive restorations and caries, an argument could be made for loss of all four first molars in this case.

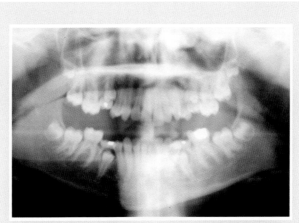

Fig. 26 Dental pantomogram of a patient with all four second deciduous molars submerging. Those which are below the contact point (upper right second deciduous molar) should probably be removed in order to aid eruption. The others should be observed

OTHER IMPACTIONS

The only other impactions to be considered in a general form are first molars. These may impact in soft tissue and it is sometimes worth considering occlusal exposure where a first molar has not erupted. This usually occurs in the upper arch and can be accepted if the oral hygiene is good with minimal caries experience. Impacted molars of this type quite frequently self correct before or during eruption of the second premolar. There may also be primary failure of eruption and if the tooth fails to move with orthodontic traction this is usually a good indication that the tooth will not move. First molars may also impact into second deciduous molars as they erupt and the options then are to try and move the molar distally with a headgear or removable appliance, to consider using separators (brass wire) to relieve the impaction or ultimately to remove the second deciduous molar if any of these methods fail to relieve the impaction.

It is clear that the biggest single contribution that can be made to the treatment of impacted teeth is to improve diagnostic skills and define care pathways with clinical protocols. Early referral does not harm, a late referral will increase the burden of care for patients and practitioners.

1. Ericson S, Kurol J. Early treatment of palatally erupting maxillary canines by extraction of the primary canine. *Eur J Orthod* 1988; **10:** 283-295.
2. Power S, Short M B E. An investigation into the response of palatally displaced canines to the removal of deciduous canines and an assessment of factors contributing to favourable eruption. *Br J Orthod* 1993; **20:** 215-223.
3. *National Clinical Guidelines.* Faculty of Dental Surgery, Royal College of Surgeons of England, 1997.

11

IN BRIEF

- The osteoblast is the pivotal cell in bone remodelling and the link between the osteoblast and osteoclast recruitment and activation is now established
- Excessive orthodontic forces causes inefficient tooth movement and adverse tissue reactions
- The mechanisms which prevent root resorption are not fully understood but it remains a consequence of any orthodontic treatment. The extent and degree of root resorption cannot be predicted but some indicators are available

Orthodontic tooth movement

D. Roberts-Harry and J. Sandy

Orthodontic tooth movement is dependent on efficient remodelling of bone. The cell-cell interactions are now more fully understood and the links between osteoblasts and osteoclasts appear to be governed by the production and responses of osteoprotegerin ligand. The theories of orthodontic tooth movement remain speculative but the histological documentation is unequivocal. A periodontal ligament placed under pressure will result in bone resorption whereas a periodontal ligament under tension results in bone formation. This phenomenon may be applicable to the generation of new bone in relation to limb lengthening and cranial-suture distraction. It must be remembered that orthodontic tooth movement will result in root resorption at the microscopic level in every case. Usually this repairs but some root characteristics apparent on radiographs before treatment begins may be indicative of likely root resorption. Some orthodontic procedures (such as fixed appliances) are also known to cause root resorption.

The histological changes which occur when forces are applied to teeth are well documented (Figs 1 and 2). Teeth appear to lie in a position of balance between the tongue and lips or cheeks. This zone is not completely neutral since tongue forces are usually slightly greater than the lips or cheeks. The periodontal ligament is thought to have an intrinsic force which has to be overcome before teeth move. A notable feature of periodontal disease, where this intrinsic force is lost, is splaying, drifting and spacing of teeth. Similarly, if there is excessive tongue activity or destruction of the lips or cheeks (as in cancrum oris) then the teeth will drift.

Very low forces are capable of moving teeth. Classically, ideal forces in orthodontic tooth movement are those which just overcome capillary blood pressure. In this situation bone resorption is seen on the pressure side and bone deposition on the tension side. Teeth rarely move in this ideal way. Usually force is not applied evenly and teeth move by a series of tipping and uprighting movements. In some areas excessive pressure results in hyalanization where the cellular component of the periodontal ligament disappears. The hyalanized zone assumes a ground glass appearance but this returns to normal once the pressure is reduced and the periodontal ligament repopulated with normal cells. In this situation a different type of resorption is seen whereby osteoclasts appear to 'undermine' bone rather than resorbing at the 'frontal' edge (Fig. 3).

Mechanically induced remodelling is not fully understood. The role of the periodontal ligament has been questioned since tooth movement can still occur even where the periodontal ligament is not functioning normally. The ligament itself undergoes remodelling and the role of matrix metalloproteinases (MMPs) together with their natural inhibitors, tissue inhibitors of metalloproteinases (TIMPs) are clearly of importance.[1]

Osteocytes (osteoblasts incorporated into mineralized bone matrix) are situated in a rigid matrix and are thus ideally positioned to detect changes in mechanical stresses. They could signal to surface lining osteoblasts and thus bone formation and indeed bone resorption may result. There is now good understanding of key mechanisms in bone resorption and formation. Bone is formed by osteoblasts which also have a role in bone resorption. It is the osteoblast which has receptors for many of the hormones and growth factors which stimulate bone turnover.

By contrast, the osteoclast which resorbs mineralised tissue, responds to very few direct hormone actions. Most of the classic agents which have direct effects on osteoclasts have inhibitory actions. For example, Calcitonin and prostaglandin E2 will inhibit osteoclasts from resorbing calcified matrices.

The recruitment and activation of osteoclasts to sites of resorption comes from the osteoblast when the latter cell is stimulated by various hormones. The signal link from osteoblasts has recently been identified as osteoprotegerin (OPG) and the ligand (OPGL). They both potently inhibit and stimulate respectively, osteoclast differentiation. Furthermore, OPGL appears to have direct effects on stimulating mature osteoclasts into activity. If OPGL is injected into mice there is an

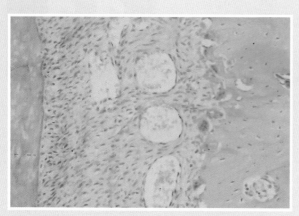

Fig. 1 Pressure side of a tooth being moved. The very vascular periodontal ligament has cementum on one side and bone on the other where frontal resorption is occurring. Osteoclasts can be seen in their lacunae resorbing bone on it's 'frontal edge'

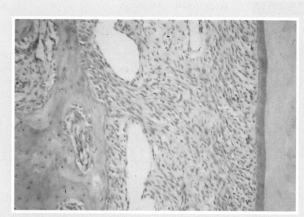

Fig. 2 This is a tension site where the bone adjacent to the periodontal ligament has surface lining osteoblasts and no sign of any osteoclasts. New bone is laid down as the tooth moves

Intermittent forces appear to move teeth and stimulate bone remodelling more efficiently than continuous forces

increase in ionised blood calcium within 1 hour. These finding have done much to unravel the final links between bone formation and resorption.

One other role that osteoblasts have in bone resorption is removal of the non-mineralised osteoid layer. In response to bone resorbing hormones, the osteoblast secretes MMPs which are responsible for removal of osteoid. This exposes the mineral layer to osteoclasts for resorption. It has been suggested that the mineral is also chemotactic for osteoclast recruitment and function.

How mechanical forces stimulate bone remodelling remains a mystery but some key facts are known. First, intermittent forces stimulate more bone remodelling than continuous forces. It is likely that during orthodontic tooth movement intermittent forces are generated because of 'jiggling' effects as teeth come into occlusal contact. Second, that the key regulatory cell in bone metabolism is the osteoblast. It is therefore relevant to examine what effects mechanical forces have on these cells. The application of a force to a cell membrane triggers off a number of responses inside the cell and this is usually mediated by second messengers. It is known that cyclic AMP, inositol phosphates and intracellular calcium are all elevated by mechanical forces. Indeed the entry of calcium to the cell may come from G-protein controlled ion channels or release of calcium from internal cellular stores. These messengers will evoke a nuclear response which will either result in production of factors responsible for osteoclast recruitment and activation, or bone forming growth factors. An indirect pathway of activation also exists whereby membrane enzymes (phospholipase A2) make substrate (arachidonic acid) available for the generation of prostaglandins and leukotrienes. These compounds have both been implicated in tooth movement.

The main theories of tooth movement are now summarised:

BIOMECHANCIAL ORTHODONTIC TOOTH MOVEMENT

This theory simply states that mechanically distorting a cell membrane activates PLA2 making arachidonic acid available for the action of cyclo and lipoxygenase enzymes. This produces prostaglandins which feed back onto the cell membrane binding to receptors which then stimulate second messengers and elicit a cell response. Ultimately, these responses will include bone being laid down in tension sites and bone being resorbed at pressure sites. It is not clear how tissues discriminate between tension and pressure. It is worth remembering that cells which are rounded up show catabolic changes whereas flattened cells (? under tension) have anabolic effects.

BONE BENDING, PIEZOELECTRIC AND MAGNETIC FORCES

There was considerable interest in piezoelectricity as a stimulus for bone remodelling during the 1960s. This arose because it was noted that distortion of crystalline structures generated small electrical charges, which potentially may have been responsible for signalling bone changes associated with mechanical forces. The interest therefore in 'electricity' and bone was considerable.

Magnets have been used to provide the force needed for orthodontic tooth movement. Classically an unerupted tooth has a magnet attached to it and a second magnet is placed on an orthodontic appliance with the poles orientated to provide an attractive force. It is unlikely that the magnetic forces alone have any actions on tissues. If magnetic fields are broken (as in pulsed electromagnetic fields) then there is some evidence that tissues will respond. It is worth making the following points about the effects of magnetic and electric fields on tooth movement:

- The periodontal ligament is unlikely to transfer forces to bone. If the periodontal ligament is disrupted, orthodontic tooth movement still occurs

- Magnetic fields alone have little, if any, effect on tissues
- Pulsed magnetic fields (which induce electric fields) can increase the rate and amount of tooth movement
- When an orthodontic force is applied, the tooth is displaced many times more than the periodontal ligament width. Bone bending must therefore occur in order to account for the tooth movement over and above the width of the periodontal ligament
- Physically distorting dry bone produces piezoelectric forces which have been implicated in tooth movement. Piezoelectric forces are those charges which develop as a consequence of distorting any crystalline structure. The magnitude of the charges is very small and there is some doubt whether they are sufficient to induce cellular change.
- It must also be remembered that in hydrated tissues, streaming potential and nerve impulses produce larger electrical fields and thus it is unlikely that piezoelectric forces alone are responsible for tooth movement.[2]

A wider application of the phenomenon of mechanically induced bone remodelling is seen where sutures are stretched. In young orthodontic patients the midline palatal suture can be split using rapid maxillary expansion techniques. The resulting tension generates new bone which fills in between the distracted maxillary shelves. A similar technique is also used to lengthen limbs. This method, known as distraction osteogenesis, can be used in any situation where it is hoped that new bone will be generated. Originally this was described in Russia where many soldiers returning from war faced the problem of non-union limb fractures. Initially attempts were made to induce new bone formation by compressing bone ends. It was only when a patient inadvertently turned the screw for compression of bone ends in the wrong direction that it was noted excessive new bone formation was seen where bone ends were distracted rather than compressed.

This may also have application in patients whose sutures fuse prematurely (craniosynostoses such as Crouzon's or Aperts Syndrome). In this situation continued growth of the brain results in a characteristic appearance of the cranium but more importantly the eyes become protuberant with possible damage to the optic nerve. Treatment involves surgically opening the prematurely fused sutures and burring out to enable normal brain growth. If distraction forces are applied prior to this early fusion then bony infill could occur at a controlled rate. The phenomenon of pressure resulting in bone loss is also seen in pathological lesions. Much work was done to examine pressures within cystic lesions and to equate this with the rate of bone destruction. It is now recognised that cytokines and bone resorbing factors produced by cystic and malignant lesions are more likely to be responsible for the associated bone resorption.

Tension results in bone formation, this can be used to generate new bone for digit lengthening or suture distraction

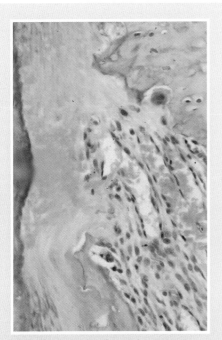

Fig. 3 This is an area of excessive pressure where the periodontal ligament has been crushed or 'hylanized' and the periodontal ligament has lost its structure. There is a large cell lying in a lacunae behind the frontal edge which is probably an area of undermining resorption

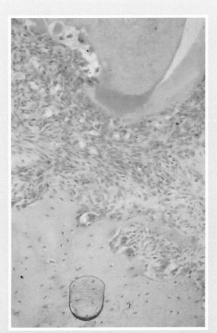

Fig. 4 Area of root resorption associated with orthodontic tooth movement. The apex of the tooth has a large excavation of the root surface and this is typical of excessive tipping forces that are placed on the apices of the teeth

ROOT RESORPTION

The ability to move teeth through bone is dependent on bone being resorbed and tooth roots remaining intact. It is highly probable that all teeth which have undergone orthodontic tooth movement exhibit some degree of microscopic root resorption (Fig. 4). Excessive root resorption is found in 3–5% of orthodontic patients. Some teeth are more susceptible than others, upper lateral incisors can, on average, lose 2 mm of root length during a course of fixed orthodontic treatment. There are specific features of appliances which can increase the risk of root resorption. The following are considered risk factors:

- Fixed appliances
- Class II elastics
- Rectangular wires
- Orthognathic surgery

There is also some evidence that the use of functional appliances appears to cause less resorption than fixed appliances and may be used to reduce increased overjet where there are recognised risks of root resorption which include pre-existing features such as:

- Short roots
- Blunt root apices
- Thin conical roots
- Root filled teeth
- Teeth which have been previously traumatised

What prevents roots from resorbing is not known but the following have been suggested:

- Cementum has anti-angiogenic properties. This means blood vessels are inhibited from forming adjacent to cementum and osteoclasts have less access for resorption.
- Periodontal ligament fibres are inserted more densely in cementum than alveolar bone and thus osteoclasts have less access to the cemental layer.
- Cementum is harder than bone and more densely mineralised.
- Cemental repair may be by a material which is intermediate between bone and cementum. These semi-bone like cells may be more responsive to systemic factors such as parathyroid hormone and thus where roots are already short (and repaired with a bone/cementum like material) the teeth are more susceptible to further root resorption.

The exact reason why roots generally do not resorb is not known but without this property it would not be possible to move teeth orthodontically. A number of reviews are available which cover bone remodelling and tooth movement in greater depth.[3,4]

1. Waddington R J, Embery G, Samuels R H. Characterization of proteoglycan metabolites in human gingival fluid during orthodontic tooth movement. *Arch Oral Biol* 1994; **39:** 361-368.
2. McDonald F. Electrical effects at the bone surface. *Eur J Orthod* 1993; **15:** 175-183.
3. Hill P A. Bone remodelling. *Br J Orthod* 1998; **25:** 101-107.
4. Sandy J R, Farndale R W, Meikle M C. Recent advances in understanding mechanically-induced bone remodelling and their relevance to orthodontic theory and practice. *Am J Orthod Dento-fac Orthop* 1993; **103:** 212-222.

IN BRIEF

● The dental specialities can collaborate with the treatment of complex cases
● Joint treatment planning is essential
● A clear treatment plan must be agreed by all parties prior to treatment starting
● Responsibility for each treatment stage must be agreed in advance
● Combined treatment can produce high quality treatment outcomes in complex cases

12

Combined orthodontic treatment

D. Roberts-Harry and J. Sandy

Dentistry is becoming more sophisticated and capable of providing much higher treatment standards than ever before. Treatments previously considered impossible can now be achieved as a direct consequence of these advances. However, this increased complexity of treatment also means that the different branches of dentistry have, as a necessity, become more and more specialised. However, it is important that the specialities collaborate in a systematic focused way to ensure the optimal treatment outcome with the minimum burden of care for the patient.

Recent advances in dentistry, coupled with patients' increased expectations and demands, means that some areas of clinical practice have become more specialised. An individual dentist is unlikely to have the necessary skills and expertise to undertake all aspects of treatment. In the management of complex cases joint planning between the orthodontist and the other dental specialities is important if a satisfactory treatment outcome is to be obtained. The dental specialities cannot work in isolation, and joint-working relationships should be fostered. Whilst orthodontists may be highly skilled in moving teeth, they are heavily dependent on other dental disciplines if optimal treatment outcomes are to be achieved in complex cases.

There are many areas in which orthodontic treatment may be of help to other dental specialities. Some of these are as follows:

● Missing teeth
● Traumatised teeth
● Periodontal problems
● Occlusal problems
● Surgical problems

MISSING TEETH

The choice in these cases is usually to recreate space for the prosthetic replacement of missing teeth, or to close the space instead.

If an upper central incisor is missing then the usual choice is to open up the space and put in some form of prosthesis. If the space is closed and the lateral incisor is placed in the central incisor site, then camouflage is difficult because of the small width of the lateral that results in an unsightly emergence angle of the crown. In cases where an upper incisor is missing, the space may need to be re-distributed. The patient in Figure 1 had a partial upper denture, and it was difficult to restore the site with a bridge because of the inclination of the upper lateral incisor and the generalised spacing in the upper labial segment. Fixed appliances were therefore used to re-distribute the space in the upper arch. In order to maintain the appearance, a bracket was fitted to a denture tooth. At the completion of treatment the patient was fitted with an upper removable retainer carrying a denture tooth. Note the proximal metal stops on the upper right central and upper left lateral incisor, to prevent a space re-opening during retention. Finally a bonded bridge restored the site.

When lateral incisors are missing the choice is not so clear-cut, and often depends on the amount of spacing the patient has, the buccal occlusion and the shape and colour of the canines. Opening the space for prosthetic replacement produces optimal aesthetics but has the disadvantage of the maintenance involved with this type of restorative treatment. Closing the space obviates the need for false teeth but this may produce a less satisfactory appearance.

Where there is considerable space, the buccal occlusion is well inter-cuspated and the canine has a pointed cusp tip then the usual treatment is to open the spaces. Closing spaces will affect the buccal occlusion, and if it is a well interdigitated Class I then this may not be the best option. The shape of the canines is

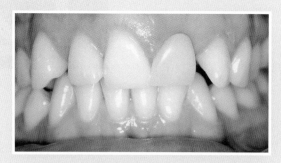

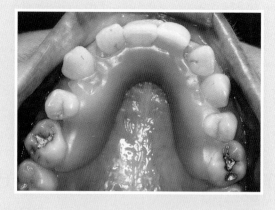

Fig.1a,b A patient with a missing upper left central incisor, which has been replaced with an inadequate denture

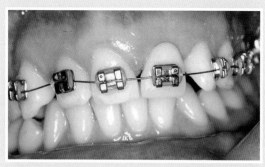

Fig. 1c A fixed appliance with a denture tooth to mask the space

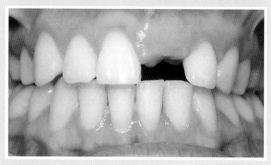

Fig. 1d The space has been redistributed

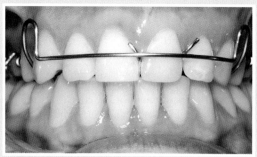

Fig. 1e A retainer with a denture tooth. Note the proximal metal stops. If these are not used there is a risk of the teeth sliding past the denture tooth.

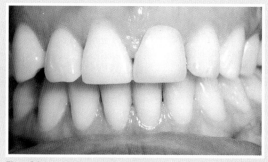

Fig. 1f A bonded bridge was placed 1 year after the removal of the fixed appliance

important because if they are pointed they will look unsightly adjacent to the central incisor. Although the tips of the teeth can be trimmed to improve their appearance, this is not always the best choice. Figure 2 shows a case with spacing in the upper arch due to developmentally absent upper lateral incisors. The upper canines have very pointed tips and it would be difficult to modify the shape of these teeth to make them resemble lateral incisors. In addition, the buccal occlusion would make space closure very difficult. Therefore, space in the upper arch was recreated to allow prosthetic replacement. An upper fixed appliance with coil springs at the upper lateral incisor sites accomplished this task. At the completion of treatment, an upper retainer with denture teeth was used to restore the missing sites. This retainer was worn for a year prior to definitive restoration with adhesive bridgework.

If the canine teeth are more amenable to masking, and the buccal occlusion is not well inter-cuspated with less spacing in the upper arch, then consideration can be given to space closure. Figure 3 shows a case where this was accomplished, again using a fixed appliance and the tips of the canines subsequently trimmed. A good aesthetic appearance was achieved, but it is worth noting the slightly different colour of the canines in relation to the central incisors. If necessary, this can then be masked with veneers. Before the decision to open or close spaces is made, consultation with a restorative dentist or the patient's GDP is a pre-requisite.

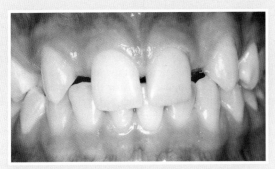

Fig. 2a A patient with missing upper lateral incisors and spacing

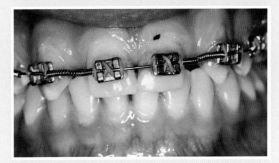

Fig.2b A fixed appliance with coil springs to re-open the spaces for the lateral incisors

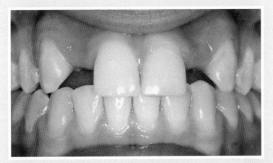

Fig. 2c Following removal of the fixed appliance

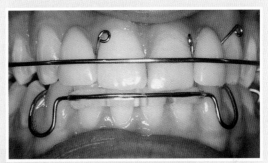

Fig. 2d A retainer with denture teeth was fitted and worn for one year prior to definitive restorative treatment

TRAUMATISED TEETH

Traumatised, fractured, intruded or avulsed teeth may sometimes benefit from an orthodontic input. Teeth, which are fractured or intruded, may need extrusion, and this can be accomplished by using a number of different appliances and techniques. Figure 4 is an example of an upper appliance being used to extrude two unerupted upper incisors as an interceptive form of treatment. The upper permanent lateral incisors had already erupted; a clear sign that something was wrong. A supernumerary tooth, preventing the eruption of the central incisors, was first removed and brackets bonded to the central incisors. A modified palatal arch was then fitted and attached to the central incisor brackets with wire ligatures. The ligatures were gently activated to extrude the teeth. Once the teeth had erupted the remaining dentition was then allowed to develop prior to definitive orthodontic treatment. A similar technique can also be used to extrude fractured roots so that post-crowns can be placed on the teeth.

If upper incisors are traumatised and have a poor prognosis it is occasionally possible to transplant teeth to restore these sites. The main principles of transplantation have been well documented by Andreasen[1] and provided these are followed, success rates in excess of 90% can be expected. Premolars are good teeth to replace upper central incisors because they often have the same width at the gingival margin as the teeth they are replacing. Figure 5 shows an

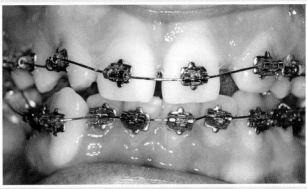

Fig. 3a Another case with missing upper lateral incisors

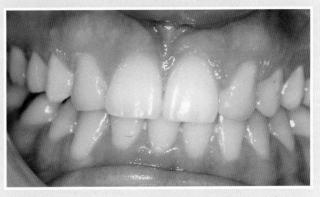

Fig. 3b Because the spaces were small these were closed up using a fixed appliance

example of a case where the upper incisors had a poor prognosis and were extracted. The lower first premolars were then transplanted into the extraction sites. Veneers were then placed on the premolars to produce a satisfactory treatment outcome. The advantage of transplantation over implants is that transplantation can be undertaken at an early age and will grow as the patient grows. If an implant were placed at this stage it would, as the child grows, become gradually submerged. There is also a risk of ridge resorption by waiting until the patient is old enough to have an implant placed. In addition the cost of transplantation is also considerably less than for implants.

PERIODONTAL PROBLEMS

With advanced periodontal disease, teeth are prone to drift producing an unsightly appearance. The teeth can be realigned orthodontically, but prior to this it is essential that all pre-existing periodontal disease is eliminated and the patient can maintain a meticulous standard of oral hygiene. If treatment is undertaken in the presence of active disease, very rapid bone loss can result.

Figure 6 shows a patient who had substantial vertical and horizontal bone loss, and as a consequence, drifting of the upper teeth had occurred, in particular the upper lateral incisor. Alignment of the teeth was achieved using fixed appliances. Near the completion of treatment a residual black triangle was left between the upper incisors. This is quite a common problem in adults and is caused by the inability of the gingival tissue to regenerate and re-form an inter-dental papilla. In order to reduce the size of the black triangle, some inter-proximal reduction was undertaken to reshape the mesial contact points of the incisors allowing the teeth to be brought more closely together. Permanent retention is needed in situations like this because the tooth will drift as soon as the appliances are removed.

OCCLUSAL PROBLEMS

Orthodontics can be used to try and produce an optimal occlusion, and there are many situations in which this can be used.[2] The occlusion can be adjusted to provide canine guidance, and eliminate non-working side interferences. In situations where anterior open bites exist, it is occasionally possible to close these down without the need to resort to surgery.[3]

Sometimes the occlusion can damage the teeth and supporting tissues. Figure 8 is an example of a patient with a unilateral cross bite extending from the upper central incisor to the terminal molar on the right hand side. This traumatic occlusion had produced substantial tooth wear. Treatment was carried out using an upper fixed appliance in conjunction with a quad helix to expand the upper arch, correct the cross-bite and align the teeth. At the completion of treatment the incisal tips were restored with composite.

SURGERY

There is a limit to how much tooth movement can be achieved, and in cases with severe skeletal discrepancies, orthodontics alone is not capable of correcting the incisor relationship, or improving facial aesthetics. In these circumstances close liaison with an oral and maxillofacial surgeon will be required. An outline of the processes involved and the orthodontist's role in orthognathic surgery has recently been reviewed.[4]

Figure 7 shows an example of a patient with a Class III skeletal pattern. There has been some dento-alveolar compensation with the lower incisors retroclined and the upper incisors proclined in an attempt to make incisal contact. There is no scope for correcting the incisor relationship further with orthodontics alone. A combined orthodontic/surgical protocol was established and the patient started treatment with fixed appliances, in order to decompensate the incisors. This made the incisor relationship and the facial profile worse. Clearly, patients need to

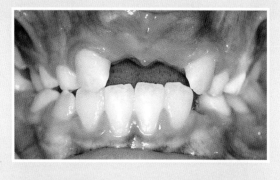

Fig. 4a The presence of a supernumerary tooth prevented the eruption of the upper central incisors

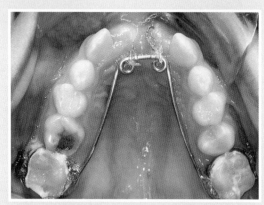

Fig. 4b The supernumerary was surgically removed and brackets bonded to the upper incisors. A modified trans-palatal bar with wire ligatures was used to extrude the teeth

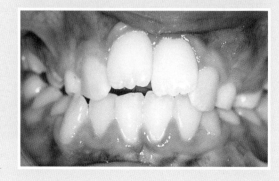

Fig. 4c Once the teeth were successfully extruded the dentition was allowed to develop prior to comprehensive treatment in the permanent dentition

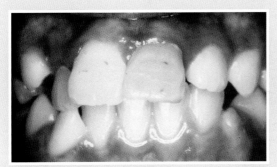

Fig. 5a Both the upper central incisors had been badly damaged after a fall

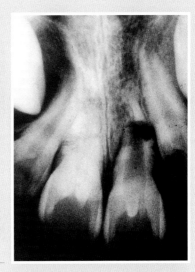

Fig. 5b A peri–apical radiograph indicated that the teeth had a hopeless prognosis

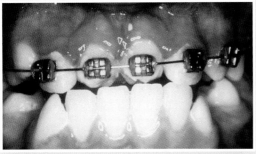

Fig. 5c The teeth were extracted and two lower premolars transplanted into the extraction sites. The teeth were then aligned with fixed appliances

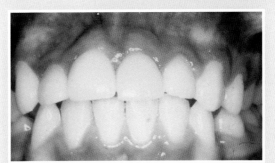

Fig. 5d At the completion of fixed appliance treatment veneers were placed on the transplanted teeth

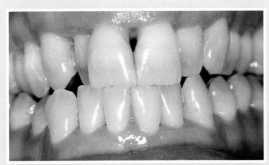

Fig. 6a The patient complained that her teeth had moved and were getting worse. She had extensive periodontal disease that needed addressing prior to any orthodontic treatment

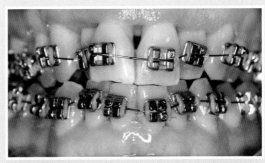

Fig. 6b Fixed appliances were then used to realign the teeth

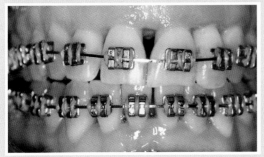

Fig. 6c A dark triangle between the anterior teeth is a common complication of treatment in adults. This is because the inter-dental papilla fails to regenerate

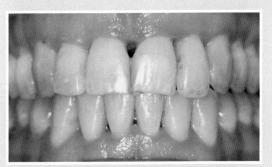

Fig. 6d Inter-proximal reduction (slenderizarition) of the contact points helped to substantially reduce the gap and improve the aesthetics

Fig. 7a–d Pre-treatment photographs of a patient with a Class III incisor relationship and skeletal pattern. The problem is beyond the scope of orthodontics alone because of the skeletal discrepancy

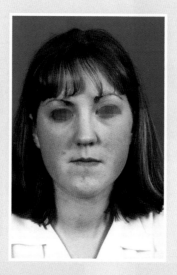
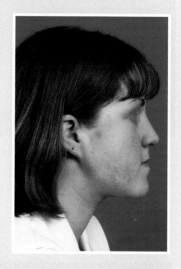

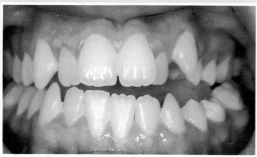
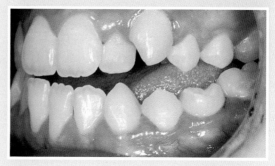

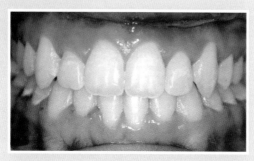
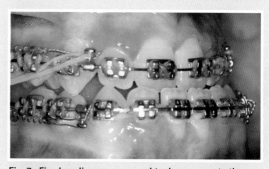

Fig. 7e Fixed appliances were used to decompensate the incisors and co-ordinate the arches prior to bi-maxillary orthognathic surgery

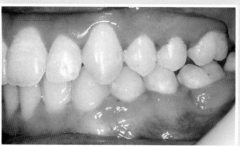

Fig. 7f–i The completed case

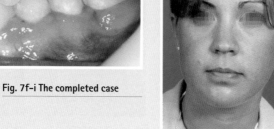
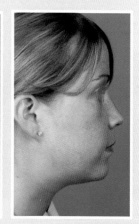

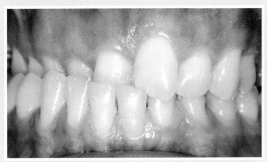
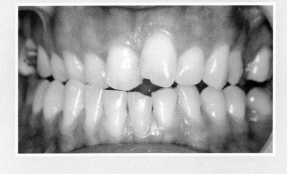

Fig. 8a,b A right–sided cross bite has produced substantial occlusal wear. This would be impossible to correct restoratively with this occlusion

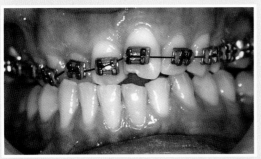

Fig. 8c An upper fixed appliance with a quad helix was used to expand the upper arch, correct the incisor relationship and align the teeth

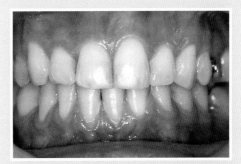

Fig. 8d At the completion of orthodontic treatment the teeth were restored with composite

be advised of this prior to the commencement of treatment. Once the incisors are decompensated and the arches co-ordinated the patient is ready for surgery. The maxilla was advanced 7 mm and the mandible set back by 6 mm, producing an overall change of 13 mm in the skeletal relationship. In addition, because the patient had a facial asymmetry, the mandible was rotated in order to correct this.

As dentistry becomes increasingly sophisticated with more treatment options available than ever before, no single specialty in dentistry can work alone to provide the full range treatment options. Some of the most interesting aspects of orthodontic treatment come from working in a combined approach with one's colleagues and it is important to recognize and respect the skills of other disciplines. Work of this nature can be amongst the most satisfying both for the clinician and the patient.

The authors thank Paul Cook for the use of figures 5(a–d)

1. Andreasen J O, Andreasen F. *Textbook and color atlas of traumatic injuries to the teeth.* 3rd ed. pp671-690. Munksgaard, Copenhagen: Mosby, 1994.
2. Davies S J, Gray R M J, Sandler P J, O'Brien K D O. Orthodontics and occlusion. *Br Dent J* 2001; **191**: 539-549.
3. Kim Y H. Anterior openbite and its treatment with multiloop edgewise archwire. *Angle Orthod* 1987; **57**: 290-321.
4. Sandy J R, Irvine G H, Leach A. Update on orthognathic surgery. *Dent Update* 2001; **28**: 337-345.

Index